HEALTH PROMOTION FOR NURSES

Health promotion is an increasingly high-profile aspect of a nurse's role – both in line with health policy and as nursing has shifted from a disease model to a health model. This textbook explores how and why health promotion works in nursing, developing a new framework for understanding the nurse's role and promoting evidence-based practice.

Drawing on empirical research and discussing existing theories of health promotion and of nursing, Stewart Piper identifies three principal approaches:

- the nurse as behaviour change agent
- the nurse as strategic practitioner
- the nurse as empowerment facilitator.

The book describes the aims, processes, impact and outcomes of health promotion interventions in nursing for each of these models and identifies criteria for evaluating the associated nursing interventions – enabling clinical judgements about effective practice.

Evidence-based examples throughout the book demonstrate the relationship between health promotion theory and pragmatic applications for nursing, and each chapter includes an introduction, learning outcomes and exercises, making this an essential book for all nursing students studying health promotion.

Stewart Piper is a Senior Lecturer in the Faculty of Health and Social Care at Anglia Ruskin University, UK. His academic and research interests include the relationship between health promotion theory and nursing practice and empowerment.

HEALTH PROMOTION FOR NURSES

THEORY AND PRACTICE

STEWART PIPER

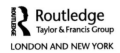

Routledge
Taylor & Francis Group

LONDON AND NEW YORK

First published 2009
by Routledge
2 Park Square, Milton Park, Abingdon, Oxon OX14 4RN

Simultaneously published in the USA and Canada
by Routledge
270 Madison Avenue, New York, NY 10016

Transferred to digital printing 2009

Routledge is an imprint of the Taylor & Francis Group, an informa business

© 2009 Stewart Piper

Typeset in Times New Roman and Futura by
Florence Production Ltd, Stoodleigh, Devon
Printed and bound in Great Britain by
CPI Antony Rowe, Chippenham, Wiltshire

British Library Cataloguing in Publication Data
A catalogue record for this book is available from
the British Library

Library of Congress Cataloging in Publication Data
Piper, Stewart, 1961–.
    Health promotion for nurses: theory and practice/Stewart Piper.
        p. cm.
    Includes bibliographical references.
    1. Health promotion.   2. Nursing.   3. Health education.   I. Title.
    RT90.3.P56 2009
    610.73 – dc22   2008035343

ISBN10: 0–415–46262–2 (hbk)
ISBN10: 0–415–46263–0 (pbk)

ISBN13: 978–0–415–46262–4 (hbk)
ISBN13: 978–0–415–46263–1 (pbk)

FOR KAREN, WILLIAM AND JOSEPH WITH LOVE

CONTENTS

CONTENTS

ACKNOWLEDGEMENTS

A number of people have provided help, support and guidance over the years. For some this has been constant and enduring, for others it has been offered at particular points. I am grateful to all, but some require individual mention. I owe a particular academic debt of thanks to Peter Brown, Dr Peter Duncan, Professor Shula Ramon, David Lewin, Dr Tessa Muncey and Professor Helen Valentine and I thank Professor Diane DeBell for her unwavering encouragement. This gratitude is extended to librarians Susan Knight and Peter Stokes for their tireless efforts in all matters related to literature searching. Finally, Routledge are thanked for granting permission to reproduce Figure 2.1 from copyright material.

Projects of this nature and duration incur considerable personal cost and I am grateful to my wife Karen, two sons William and Joseph and my Mum for their love and tolerance. I apologise to them for the time and effort invested in this book that could have otherwise been spent as a husband, father and son.

INTRODUCTION

For some time, health promotion has been a central feature of general health policy within the developed world. For example, in the UK *Saving Lives: our healthier nation* (Department of Health 1999a), *Choosing Health* (Department of Health 2004a) and *Better Information, Better Choices, Better Health* (Department of Health 2004b) emphasise health promotion as a health service priority. The former states its intention to save 300,000 lives by 2010 and add years to life and years free from illness. *The NHS Plan* (Department of Health 2000) has prevention as its ninth core principle and refers to keeping people healthy and reducing inequalities in health.

The US Department of Health and Human Services *Healthy People 2010* (2000) strategy focuses on disease prevention, health promotion objectives and public health priorities. The sub-title of the strategy announces that it is about 'understanding and improving health'. *The Evaluation of the Eleven Primary Health Care Nursing Innovation Projects* report (Primary Health Care Nursing Innovation Evaluation Team 2007) in New Zealand refers to Primary Health Organisations (PHOs) providing preventive health services. *The Primary Health Care Strategy* of New Zealand (Ministry of Health 2001: 13) states that 'improving health involves health promotion' while Canada has *The Integrated Pan-Canadian Healthy Living Strategy* (Secretariat for the Intersectoral Healthy Living Network 2005).

The UK *NHS Plan* (2000) also refers to the disempowering nature of the hierarchical and paternalistic patient/health care professional relationship and the need to empower patients. The latter theme has been pursued further by the UK Department of Health (2001a) introducing the concept of the expert patient and the introduction of patient advice and liaison services (PALS) (Department of Health 2002). *The NHS Plan*, *The Pan-Canadian Healthy Living Strategy* and the US *Healthy People 2010* also include reference to partnership working with individuals and communities.

More specifically, increasing emphasis has been given to the illness prevention and health promotion aspect of the nurse's role in the UK (Department of Health 1989, 1993, 1999b). The debate was given impetus in 1992 by *The Health of the Nation* (HoN), the government strategy for health in England (Department of Health 1992). The HoN placed health promotion explicitly on the nursing agenda in general and on some specialist areas of practice in particular. For example, emergency care nurses came under close scrutiny as accidents were one of the five key areas of the strategy; with the HoN (1993) requiring emergency departments to help reduce ill-health, disability and death via their prevention role.

The UK Nursing and Midwifery Council also highlight the important role of health promotion in nursing. It is a standard of proficiency for pre-registration nursing education (2004a) and specialist community public health nurses (2004b) while the code of professional conduct (2004c) states that the health of individual patients/clients and the community must be protected and supported.

Ditto the education programme standards for the registered nurse scope of practice of the Nursing Council of New Zealand (2005), which refers to supporting people to manage their health and includes health promotion in the content of the criteria for standard three. The American Nurses Association (2007) also call for nursing to engage more with the promotion of health and the prevention of disease, illness and disability at group and population levels and from primary, secondary and tertiary perspectives.

In addition, in the UK competence in illness prevention and health promotion is a feature of Nurse Training Rule 18 (1) of *The Nurses, Midwives and Health Visitors Rules Approval Order* (Statutory Instruments 1983, No. 873), and the inception of Project 2000 nurse training shifted the curriculum emphasis from a disease model to a health model. The requirement was for the Common Foundation Programme element to focus on health and not illness (UKCC 1986). Parallel developments impinging on nursing include the call for an expansion of the public health role of some practitioners (Department of Health 1999b), local health strategies in the UK, and the World Health Organization (WHO) Health Promoting Hospitals (1991a,

1997) initiative. Health education and health promotion also feature prominently in research findings and internal debate in the nursing literature. Indeed Macleod Clark and Webb (1985) heralded health promotion as a basis for nursing practice over 20 years ago, and this is consistent with Beattie's (1991) contention that health care professionals have increasingly claimed that health promotion forms the foundation for their work.

NURSING

Various authors and organisations have sought to define nursing. For Henderson (1970), nursing is concerned to help people to engage in activities that improve health or aid recovery and to move to a position where they are free from the need for nursing interventions. Benner and Wrubel (1989) talk about the importance of caring to the role of the nurse while Benner (1983) identified seven domains of practice when researching what defines expert nursing in acute care settings. Of particular relevance here is the teaching–coaching domain, which is about helping patients understand and develop control of their illness and adapt their lifestyle accordingly. More recently the International Council of Nurses (2004) has defined the scope of nursing practice by the criteria in Box I.1.

The Royal College of Nursing of the UK (2003) are similarly concerned with informing, educating and advising to help people understand and manage their disease or disability, and advocating for patients. They add that nursing involves promoting health and preventing disease, illness, injury, and disability.

The Nursing and Midwifery Council (2004c) of the UK support the latter and stress that all patients and clients have a right to accurate, truthful and easily understandable information about their

---

BOX I.1 THE SCOPE OF NURSING PRACTICE INCLUDES:

- the implementation and evaluation of nursing care;
- advocacy;
- supervision and delegation;
- leading, managing, teaching, researching;
- health policy development.

(International Council of Nurses 2004)

health. The Royal College of Nursing highlights the need for partnership working between nurses and patients and their relatives and carers, while *Mosby's Medical, Nursing, & Allied Health Dictionary* (2002) refers to nursing as promoting, maintaining and restoring health based on humanitarian and ethical principles.

It is clear then that health promotion is seen by policy makers and the nursing profession itself as a key role of the nurse, and Novak (1988) and The Royal College of Nursing (2003) contend that this can be traced back to Florence Nightingale. Nightingale noted how some limited nursing to administering medication or tending wounds but had the vision to see that nursing needs to address:

> fresh air, light, warmth, cleanliness, quiet, and the proper selection and administration of diet – all at the least expense of vital power to the patient.
>
> (Nightingale 1860: 3)

What is sometimes less clear is what government health policies and nursing policy and strategies mean by health promotion and how it fits with nursing. In addition, despite the contemporary emphasis on health promotion both in general and within nursing, and with copious literature on health promotion and nursing readily accessible, the emphasis tends toward what Whitehead (2005a) describes as traditional, biomedically focused practice with a narrow range of disease-related behavioural outcomes. He contends that there has been little progress or reform of health promotion in nursing in the last two decades. This position is compounded by a dearth of specific, robust, tested health promotion theory to guide nursing intervention at either clinical, community or strategic and organisational levels, and scant evidence of critical appraisal of that which does exist. Fundamental questions then, about purpose, fit with practice, and scrutiny of the different theoretical approaches and what they mean for nursing remain as much an underdeveloped area now as in previous years.

HISTORICAL CONTEXT

The 1970s heralded a shift in thinking as it became increasingly apparent that health policy needed to move beyond a medical and clinical focus to improve the health of populations (Naidoo and Wills 2000). The landmark Lalonde Report (1974), *A New Perspective on the Health of Canadians*, advanced a new way of conceptualising health. Although in the light of contemporary thinking it seems remarkable that up to this point health policy had been so narrow, Lalonde highlighted that health services are not the only determinant of health. Biology, the environment and lifestyle are equally important influences and together they constitute the 'health field concept' (Box I.2). As Parish (1995) points out, Lalonde stated that the absence of a framework had hitherto prevented a comprehensive analysis of the influences on health and a more thorough conceptualisation of the issues.

The Lalonde Report was followed in the UK by the publication of *Prevention and Health: everybody's business* (Department of Health 1976). In line with Lalonde, the policy focus shifted from treatment towards prevention. For Parish (1995), it did not entirely engage with the notion that health is determined by the wider health field and as a way to prevent disease it emphasised individual lifestyle choices and responsibility and an associated ideology (Naidoo and Wills 2000).

The above was accompanied by a significant broadening of policy by the World Health Organization. *The Declaration of Alma-Ata* (WHO 1978) reaffirmed the WHO belief in the physical, mental and social dimensions of health and that the wellbeing of people requires social and economic interventions to accompany the activities of the health sector. It also stressed that people have a right to participate individually and collectively in the planning and implementation of health care. This has been accompanied by a better understanding of the relationship between poor health and deprivation, i.e. inequalities in health in the UK (Townsend *et al.* 1988; Acheson 1998).

From the middle of the 1980s, further conferences and charters continued to advance health promotion as a movement for social and political change (Jones and Douglas 2000). In 1984 the WHO outlined the principles and subjects for health promotion. The focus was on the health of populations – life context and health determinants rather than on disease – the need to utilise a range of methods for public participation and for getting health professionals, particularly those

---

BOX I.2 THE HEALTH FIELD CONCEPT

- biology;
- environment;
- lifestyle;
- health care organisation.

(Lalonde 1974)

working in primary health care, for example community public health nurses, to enable health promotion. The *Ottawa Charter* (WHO 1986) championed equity in health.

This particular historical and policy context is reflected in the debate surrounding, and the generation of, health education and health promotion frameworks in the 1980s, culminating in the UK in an edition of the *Health Education Journal* (1990) devoted entirely to this topic. They are mostly what Bunton and Macdonald (1992) refer to as a reaction to the traditional medical model and represent a dawning recognition of, and disenchantment and crisis of spirit with, the limited effect of the traditional health-related behavioural focus of health education (Parish 1995; Rawson 2002).

The frameworks also reflect a shift in the use of terminology from health education to health promotion. For Beattie (1991), this was initiated principally by the WHO (1978) and by the Canadian Public Health Association in the early 1970s. It sparked a passionate debate in the UK over definitions and a demarcation dispute over the relationship between health education and health promotion (Beattie 1991; Tones and Tilford 1994). In addition, the frameworks reflect the classic debate about the extent to which health is the sole responsibility of the individual and how far it is a collective responsibility that requires a community and societal response that raged during the 1970s and 1980s (Parish 1995).

There are no definitive answers as to why the frameworks debate largely evanesced in the early 1990s. One potential explanation alluded to by Rawson (2002) is the new epistemology of practice for health care professionals initiated during the 1980s based on reflection, the codifying of experiences and from these generating practice theory and related goals for intervention. Nevertheless, although this discussion has mostly moved on in the health promotion literature, little of this order has taken place within nursing and a review of the former is necessary as that which has taken place within or for nursing derives from this general debate.

THEORETICAL RATIONALE FOR THIS BOOK

Agreement over a unifying framework or model for conceptualising health promotion theory and practice in general remains elusive (Naidoo and Wills 2000; Tones and Tilford 2001). Despite the frameworks and models developed or synthesised by Coutts and Hardy (1985), Davis (1995), Pender (1996), Kuss *et al.* (1997), Piper and Brown (1998a), Piper (2000, 2004, 2007a, 2007b), Whitehead (2001a),

Gonser and McGuiness (2001) and Kiger (2004) this is also the position in nursing. This conceptual confusion is exacerbated by the plethora of competing frameworks of health promotion designed to help translate theory into practice. These have been generated by copious authors, mostly from outside of nursing, and ostensibly suggest a wealth of intervention strategies. In reality, and despite varied nomenclature and apparent dichotomies, many of these are merely minor variations on the same themes, cover the same terrain, reflect the same aims, modes of intervention and outcomes and seem interchangeable.

An expansion of the health promotion role of nurses requires a repertoire of approaches, a robust means of classifying these and a sound evidence-based theory and practice relationship. However, in an evidence-based culture, the issue for nursing is how to select a framework that can be used as a basis for theorising and to classify, guide and plan a range of health promotion interventions in nursing. The difficulty with selection is further compounded by the eclectic theory base of health promotion that, like nursing (Ellis 1968), has been generated by primary feeder disciplines such as psychology and sociology (Brown and Margo 1978; Frankish and Green 1994; Freudenberg et al. 1995; Bunton and MacDonald 2002). This has prevented the development of an identifiable body of health promotion knowledge and methods resembling discipline status around which practitioners can unite (Rawson 2002).

The rationale for the book, then, is the need to reconcile the competing conceptual frameworks and claims to the theory base of health promotion and to illuminate the divergent and complementary areas for nursing. The rationale includes the need to end the directionless debate on the relative merits of the various health promotion frameworks and the models within these. Rather, an examination and analysis of the theoretical foundations, content and methods are required to establish their core theoretical elements (Rawson 2002). Further to this, there is a need for criteria to be identified that will enable systematic evaluation, critical appraisal and delineation between the health promotion frameworks. The resultant knowledge can then be used in the selection and validation of a robust structure by nurses for individual, collective, strategic and organisational health promotion.

Thus, this book advances and discusses in detail a health promotion framework developed specifically for any and all branches of general and public health nursing. Reference is made to the methods and findings used to generate and test the framework together with an outline of its relative merits in relation to competing frameworks and why it is fit for purpose. In examining and analysing the foundations, content and methods of health promotion to establish its core theory base (Rawson 2002) it explores the relationship between health promotion theory and pragmatic applications for nursing practice and uses a range of examples to illustrate the links. It also identifies criteria for systematic evaluation of the models within the framework to enable clinical judgements for health promotion nursing practice.

The unique exploration and synthesis of the theoretical basis of health promotion and ways to operationalise this for nursing to help reduce the theory practice gap is achieved in the following ways:

1   By analysing the core theory base (Rawson 2002) of nursing and health promotion and establishing their relationship. This will include defining nursing, health, health education, health promotion, health development and public health, discussing their differences and highlighting the need to adopt everyday terminology for nursing practice consistent with other disciplines and health policy.

2   By developing further a health promotion framework (Piper 2007a) constructed specifically for nursing comprising three models:

   •   the nurse as behaviour change agent;
   •   the nurse as empowerment facilitator (individual and community action perspectives);
   •   the nurse as strategic health promotion practitioner.

3   By outlining the relative merits of the above in relation to competing frameworks and why it is fit for purpose, together with a critique of the socio-political ideology that underpins each model within the framework and their degree of fit with existing theory.

4   By illustrating the relationship between health promotion theory and pragmatic applications for nursing using evidence-based examples for each model within the framework.

5   By illustrating the aims, processes, impact and evaluatory criteria and outcomes of health promotion interventions in nursing for each model within the framework to enable clinical judgements about effectiveness for practice.

However, in focusing on nursing this book is not a systematic review of health promotion programmes in general or of the related literature. The latter, while drawn from a range of sources, will be used specifically to substantiate all aspects of the framework, its inherent models and related discussion and to support the theorising and assertions of the book.

The following nine chapters then include an introduction, learning outcomes and learning triggers to accommodate distance learning focusing on theory and practice and their relationship. To facilitate conceptual understanding, and to contextualise and map out the theory base of health promotion in nursing a framework based on the work of Beattie (1991), Piper and Brown (1998a) and Piper (2000, 2007a, 2007b) forms the core of the book.

The framework comprising the nurse as behaviour change agent, the nurse as strategic practitioner and the nurse as empowerment facilitator models, derives from themes and deviant/paradigm cases generated in a qualitative study (Piper 2004), from published work and conference presentations by the author. The research examined the relationship between hospital nursing practice and health promotion theory. However, as a deviant/paradigm case the nurse as strategic practitioner was not a saturated theme and this, together with some of the example indicators of practice in the book for the other health promotion models within the framework, stems from constructive theorising and published sources to help illuminate the debate. As such, all require the tests of fit and transferability to be applied by the reader. The content of the chapters is summarised below.

PART 1: THEORY

There has been considerable debate over the meaning given to health education and health promotion and various authors have attempted to settle the theoretical disputes regarding the convergence and divergence between the two and define these concepts. Problems with defining their meaning have been compounded by the introduction of health development and a widening of the definition of public health. Thus, it is particularly important for the purpose of conceptual clarification to discuss the meaning of health education and health promotion and give a flavour of chronological development because of the need to ensure a high degree of fit between the meaning offered in the mainstream literature and policy documents and in nursing.

Chapter 1 then, defines health, health education, health promotion, primary, secondary, tertiary and quaternary health promotion, health development, health improvement and public health. The intention is not to provide an exhaustive critique of these concepts but to outline

9

the basic connections between existing theory, nursing and the language of discourse and the need for nursing to adopt contemporary language for practice if it is to make a meaningful contribution to the debate.

Chapter 2 provides definitions of theory, model and framework and delineates the relationship between them. It advances the assessment (theory testing) criteria used to gauge the theoretical rigour, breadth and depth of health promotion frameworks, identifies what makes a theoretically robust structure and outlines an exemplar from outside of nursing. Reference is also made to ideologically compatible models of health and cultural bias to develop further the analysis of the relationship between the health promotion models within the framework and to highlight their socio-political foundations. The exemplar health promotion framework is also juxtaposed with those replicating its format or integrating explicit socio-political models to help illustrate its robustness in relation to wider social theory. The benchmark criteria and framework is used to validate, develop and synthesise the proposed framework of the book and is offered as a tool for operational use by nurses to gauge its 'fitness for practice' and the credentials of competing frameworks.

Chapter 3 presents and reviews the general (i.e. from outside of nursing) frameworks of health promotion from a historical and chronological perspective to help illustrate how the debate and the construction of these devices evolved and developed. The methodology used to guide the process; the rationale for the sequence of the review; and the context of the debate is also outlined. The purpose of the review is to sketch out and consider structures that might challenge and force a reconsideration of Beattie's (1991), Piper and Brown's (1998a) and Piper's (2000, 2004, 2007a, 2007b) work that form the foundation of the health promotion framework for nursing and the basis of the book. In effect this aspect of the literature review constitutes additional, and a form of triangulated, theory testing. The comprehensive review includes a range of frameworks however described that include two or more models of health education or health promotion.

Although a wealth of published work on health promotion adorns the nursing literature, its focus is primarily pragmatic and concerned with 'doing'. Health promotion might be espoused as a fundamental part of nursing, and models and frameworks might be mentioned, but detailed description of their philosophical foundations and how to operationalise them is underdeveloped. Research on the knowledge, understanding and health promotion practice of nurses is also limited.

Thus, Chapter 4 reviews the frameworks developed or advanced for use by nurses to determine the existence of theoretical constructions that can challenge and force a reconsideration of the framework advanced by the book. In addition, the studies undertaken and articles written on health promotion and nursing and health promotion and nurse education are reviewed to reflect both the stage of theory development within nursing and the status afforded health promotion theory and practice by nursing.

In light of the absence of a unifying framework for classifying health promotion theory and practice in nursing, Chapter 5 encapsulates the uniqueness of the book in providing a detailed explanation of the framework generated for general and public health nursing designed to help address this gap. The chapter discusses the structure of the framework, theory derivation and synthesis and previews its inherent models. A framework of evaluation categories and examples of associated indicators for each model is outlined and a rationale justifying why the health promotion framework has been advanced as the structure of choice and why it is fit for purpose are included. This chapter then provides the foundation for exploring the relationship between the health promotion models (the nurse as behaviour change agent, the nurse as empowerment facilitator and the nurse as strategic practitioner) within the framework and practice in subsequent chapters.

11

PART 2: PRACTICE

Chapter 6 provides a detailed explanation of the first of the three models within the health promotion framework entitled 'The Nurse as Behaviour Change Agent'. It includes a discussion on the nature of behaviour change and modus operandi of this model in relation to top-down, nurse and expert-led practice, the medical model, compliance and associated socio-political values, i.e. the ideological premise of this model. It focuses on indicators and practical (i.e. not ideological/ theoretical) examples of the health promotion aims, processes, impact and evaluation criteria and outcomes of this traditional model for nursing practice to demonstrate the theory–practice relationship and help bridge the theory–practice gap.

Chapter 7 provides a detailed explanation of the nurse as empowerment facilitator model from an individual action perspective. It includes a discussion on the locus of control and modus operandi of this model in relation to bottom-up, individual nurse–patient partnership-based practice, advocacy, its humanistic premise, adherence/concordance and associated socio-political values, i.e. the ideological premise of this model. It focuses on indicators and practical (i.e. not ideo-logical/theoretical) examples of the health promotion aims, processes, impact and evaluation criteria and outcomes of this contemporary model for nursing practice to demonstrate the theory–practice relationship and help bridge the theory–practice gap.

Chapter 8 provides a detailed explanation of the nurse as empower-ment facilitator model from a community/collective action perspective. It includes a discussion on the locus of control and modus operandi of this model in relation to bottom-up practitioner/community partnership-based practice. The focus is on socio-political processes in the form of community development, social capital and capacity building and thus 'new' public health. The radical humanistic premise and associated socio-political values, i.e. the ideological premise of this model, are also clarified. It is accompanied by indicators and practical (i.e. not ideological/theoretical) examples of the health promotion aims, processes, impact and evaluation criteria and outcomes of this contemporary model of public health practice for nurses to demonstrate the theory–practice relationship and help bridge this gap.

Chapter 9 provides a detailed explanation of the nurse as strategic practitioner model. It includes a discussion on the locus of control and modus operandi of this model in relation to top-down, strategic, organisational and 'managerialist' (Beattie 1991: 187) interventions and associated socio-political values, i.e. the ideological premise of this model. The concept of health-promoting hospitals and related indicators and practical (i.e. not ideological/theoretical) examples of the health promotion aims, processes, impact and evaluation criteria and outcomes of this setting's approach for nursing practice are used to demonstrate the theory–practice relationship and help bridge the theory–practice gap. The conclusion summarises the discussion and considers the original contribution the book makes to conceptualising health promotion for nursing and for pragmatic application to 'real world' practice, and suggests in brief a way forward for nursing in terms of implications for practice, further research and education.

Given the above, the intention of this book is not to provide an exhaustive account or the final word on health promotion per se, but to emphasise the benefits of a conceptual framework to explore the relationship between health promotion theory and nursing practice. The intention is to move the debate beyond any narrow or traditional view of health promotion as simply a form of information or advice giving, and highlight the need for a repertoire of approaches in the modern arena of health care and nursing.

PART 1

THEORY

CONCEPT ANALYSIS AND THE LANGUAGE OF THEORY AND PRACTICE

INTRODUCTION

Consistent with the absence of consensus over a unifying framework for classifying health promotion theory and practice, there has also been considerable debate over the demarcation points and meaning given to health, health education and health promotion. Over the years attempts have been made to settle the theoretical disputes regarding the convergence and divergence between the latter two in particular and to define these concepts (for example, the UK Ministry of Health 1964; Keyes 1972; Anderson 1984; Fisher *et al.* 1986; Tones and Tilford 1994; Naidoo and Wills 2000; Tones and Tilford 2001; Tones 2001; Tones and Green 2004). However, it has not been a straightforward process. For example, Cribb (1993) found health promotion confusing because of the apparent lack of boundaries and Tannahill (1985) felt that because health education was used in different ways it was a meaningless concept. Thus, both the general and the nursing literature have found health promotion to be a contested and, at times, an ill-defined concept. Some of the definitions represent little more than broad generalisation and some authors fail to set conceptual boundaries and imply that health promotion is any activity that improves health.

Whereas for Cribb and Duncan (2001) this lack of clarity and convergence over the definition of health education and health promotion persists, for Bunton and Macdonald (2002) and Whitehead (2007a) there has been movement toward a consensus over the meaning of health promotion. These conceptual disputes have been compounded by the introduction of competing contemporary terminology, such as health development/improvement and a widening of the definition of public health. In addition, Piper (2004, 2008), when researching the meaning nurses gave to health education and health promotion and how these fitted with existing language, theory and practice, found the understanding and definition of the concepts by participants were inconsistent with the mainstream literature and contemporary health and social policy. They reflected a more traditional understanding of the term; thus lacking a modern feel and any socio-political role was overlooked.

Hence, it is important for the purpose of clarification to explore the meaning of these concepts in the general and nursing literature and policy documents, to give a flavour of their chronological development and consider these in relation to the concept of nursing theory and philosophies to identify their relationship. For Berg and Sarvimäki (2003), vague conceptualisation and the lack of a distinctive health promotion nursing focus means that such an exercise is required.

The identification of what constitutes a health promoting nurse and what this means for practice (Robinson and Hill 1998) for this book starts here. This chapter, taking and developing work from Piper's (2004) unpublished study, defines health education and health promotion (including primary, secondary, tertiary and quaternary) and the related concepts of health, public health, health development and

---

LEARNING OUTCOMES

By reading this chapter, and completing the learning triggers at the end, the reader should have a better critical understanding of:

- health as a contested concept;
- the relationship between disease and illness;
- the concept of health education;
- the concept of health promotion;
- the relationship between health education and health promotion;
- the relationship between health education, health promotion and nursing;
- primary, secondary and tertiary health promotion;
- the relationship between health promotion and nurse education;
- the concepts of public health, health development and health improvement.

THEORY

health improvement. The intention is not to provide an exhaustive critique of these concepts, as topics of this magnitude require broad academic debate to do them justice, but to outline the basic connections between them, and place in context the language of theory, policy, debate and practice for nursing.

HEALTH

Health is a contested concept. In other words, as Ewles and Simnett (1999) point out, it is different for different people and may be viewed on a continuum of subjective perceptions. These range from health being perceived as an absence of illness (medical model negative conception of health (Naidoo and Wills 2000)); having a strong constitution with the ability to fight off infection and disease; to positive expressions of mental health such as having a high self-esteem and feeling empowered. Illness is also a subjective experience, i.e. how a person feels and the signs and symptoms may be scientifically validated as disease (feels ill, has disease) by objective medical diagnosis, or disease status may be denied (no disease diagnosed despite the subjective experience of feeling ill). Individuals may also feel well with or without disease (Box 1.1). Personal perceptions of health, illness and disease are influenced by such factors as social class, cultural experiences, age and gender. These factors, together with genetic predisposition, lifestyle and environment are also important determinants of mortality and morbidity with the quality of personal relationships and social networks (social capital) as possible additional contributory factors (Kawachi *et al.* 1997).

17

BOX 1.1 THE RELATIONSHIP BETWEEN DISEASE AND ILLNESS

- feels ill, disease objectively (i.e. medically by doctor, nurse, etc.) diagnosed;
- feels ill but no objective diagnosis;
- feels well but has undetected disease;
- feels well and no disease.

(Naidoo and Wills 2000)

The key elements of the WHO (1998a) definition from the 1948 constitution state that health is a holistic and multi-dimensional concept. It is more than simply the absence of disease and:

- has physical, social and mental dimensions;
- is a resource for individuals to lead a productive social and economic life, i.e. as Seedhouse (1986) puts it, health provides the foundations for achievement in life rather than being an end in itself.

The WHO *Ottawa Charter* (1986) highlights the relationship between socio-economic conditions, the environment and both health and health-related behaviour and contends that the following conditions (Box 1.2) need to be in place before health (and thus health education/promotion outcomes) can be attained.

HEALTH EDUCATION

In 1964, the UK Ministry of Health struggled with the meaning of health education and this set the tone for subsequent discussion. They concluded that its function was to promote mental and physical health through information and instruction and to persuade people to resist using glamorous health-damaging products. They identified four categories of health education as follows:

- specific action (for example, immunisation and vaccination);
- habit and attitude change (for example, healthy eating);
- education on the appropriate use of health services;
- support for community action (for example, clean air, fluoridation).

The latter contrasts with the WHO (1954, 1969) definitions, which more closely resemble the second and third of the Ministry of Health (1964) categories. In particular, emphasis was given to persuading individuals to take action and accept the responsibility for health

---

BOX 1.2 WHO *OTTAWA CHARTER* (1986) PREREQUISITES FOR HEALTH

- peace;
- adequate economic resources;
- food and shelter;
- stable eco-system;
- sustainable resource use.

improvement (WHO 1954) and later (WHO 1969) to improve their environment in line with priorities determined by health professionals.

Despite the contested views, the general tenor of many of the definitions (for example, Griffiths 1972; Horner 1980; Baric 1982, 1985; WHO 1983; Tannahill 1985; Fisher *et al.* 1986; Nutbeam 1986; O'Donnell 1989; Downie *at al.* 1990; Tones 1990; Bunton and Macdonald 1992; WHO 1993; Naidoo and Wills 2000; Tones and Tilford 2001; Tones 2001) accord with the sub-themes of the Ministry of Health (1964). Health education aims to change beliefs, attitudes and health-related behaviour on risk factors and promote healthy lifestyles to prevent mortality and morbidity. For Baric (1982, 1985), Nutbeam (1986), Tones (1990), Bunton and Macdonald (1992) and Tones and Tilford (2001) the educational methods of health education aim to improve knowledge and understanding including on illness. Many of these interventions are based on the assumption that individuals are in a position to choose the healthy option (Minkler 1989) and reflect a top-down, expert-determined agenda where success is measured by compliance levels (Naidoo and Wills 2000). Health education is thus defined by Tones and Tilford (2001: 30) in a traditional and narrow educational way as:

> any intentional activity that is designed to achieve health or illness related learning, i.e. some relatively permanent change in an individual's capability or disposition. Effective health education may, thus, produce changes in knowledge and understanding or ways of thinking; it may influence or clarify values; it may bring about some shift in belief or attitude; it may facilitate the acquisition of skills; it may even effect changes in lifestyle or behaviour.

The limitations of this definition are acknowledged, with the literature including encouraging action on, or raising awareness about health and social policy, legislation and environmental factors and their impact on health as part of health education. It is also concerned to develop life-skills and clarify personal values (Tones 1990), equip people with the skills to manage health problems before seeking assistance from health services (Baric 1982, 1985) and to get people to use those services appropriately (Tones 1997).

For others (Griffiths 1972; WHO 1983), health education creates channels for the identification and expression of community needs or is a two-way and empowering process that embraces community development (Tannahill 1985). Greenberg (1978), Tones (1981, 1986,

1997) and Naidoo and Wills (2000) also have empowerment, and Naidoo and Wills (2000) education for informed choice, as core values of health education, but the focus is on individuals.

The WHO (1983) were critical of the top-down and paternal medical model and the almost patronising and victim-blaming tone of some of these definitions of health education. Brown and Margo (1978) also advance that although in theory health education can be a force for change, in practice ideological forces and the desire for increased professional status anchor the interventions of practitioners firmly in the established conservative health-care delivery system. A situation that still persists in nursing (Whitehead 2005a). For Brown and Margo (1978), this undermines any real contribution to progressive social development, community empowerment or an assault on the social determinants of health and disease, and contributes to maintaining the social status quo.

The above was counteracted by the WHO (1991b) who defined health education, using the type of language and terminology that has come to be associated with them, as intervention to help people be in control of their health behaviour and factors that influence health status. This clearly builds on and broadens earlier definitions and the document advances that community and societal action for equitable health, and advocacy on issues of public policy for health and empowerment are part of health education.

HEALTH PROMOTION

A starting point for defining health promotion has to be the WHO (1986) *Ottawa Charter*, as prior to this there had been little effort to establish a consensus. The WHO (1986) definition below builds on their earlier established concepts and principles of health promotion (WHO 1984). This contends that health promotion unifies change in the ways and conditions of living, mediates between people and their

---

BOX 1.3 HEALTH PROMOTION METHODS

- communication;
- education;
- legislation;
- community development.

(WHO 1986)

environments and combines personal choice with social responsibility. Although it does include promoting positive health behaviour and disseminating health information, the *Ottawa Charter* widened the debate by emphasising a population approach, a focus on social context, the cause of disease and the need to employ a range of methods (Box 1.3).

The *Ottawa Charter* (WHO 1986) espoused the need for public participation and for health professionals – particularly those working in primary health care – to enable health promotion. Its ubiquitous definition of health promotion has come to be seen as somewhat idealistic with unattainable goals, such as, for example, complete well-being. Health promotion is defined as:

> the process of enabling people to increase control over and to improve their health. To reach a state of complete physical, mental and social well-being, an individual or group must be able to identify and to realise aspirations, to satisfy needs, and to change or cope with the environment . . . health promotion is not just the responsibility of the health sector, but goes beyond healthy lifestyle to well-being.
>
> (WHO 1986: 1)

21

In outlining prerequisites for health, the *Ottawa Charter* calls for equity in health, and healthy alliances and partnerships between relevant organisations. Health promotion extends to building healthy public policy, creating supportive environments, strengthening community action and social networks, developing personal links and reorienting health services. The significance of this was in representing a departure from the medical model to a socio-political position advocating the shift of power from bureaucracies to people (Green and Raeburn 1988). It thus widened and redefined the concept of healthy public policy (Jones 1997).

Like the WHO (1993), Nutbeam's (1986) definition of health promotion concurs with the WHO (1984, 1986) but both add that it should include increasing control over the determinants of health. He draws on the principle of health promotion engaging with the community and everyday life context of people and mediating between them and their environment. They should be active participants in needs assessment and interventions on the determinants of health, and this should be part of the process of partnership between the community and public services.

At one level, health promotion is about promoting healthy lifestyles and life-skills for individuals (Anderson 1983; Fisher *et al.* 1986; Nutbeam 1986; Green and Raeburn 1988; WHO 1993) or promoting, maintaining and improving health in individuals and communities. At another, it is concerned to influence socio-economic and environmental policy for collective health gain (Baric 1985; Rutten 1995). Noak (1987) talks of integrating these policies with economic, employment and health policy and legislation and occupational health but Fisher *et al.* (1986) see legislative and public policy interventions as a means to support the adoption of health-related behaviour. Green and Raeburn (1988) take a different line in advancing that health promotion needs, including those that stem from these latter factors, can be devolved to people as long as they are equipped with the information, skills and financial and organisational wherewithal.

The starting point for Tones (1990) and Tones and Tilford (2001: 9) is that health promotion is deliberate and planned 'micro', 'meso' and 'macro' intervention to promote health and manage disease. It can be encapsulated using the domains of the health field concept of Lalonde (see Box 1.4).

A key feature of health promotion is social policy, i.e. legal, fiscal (financial) and environmental interventions. In an earlier article Tones (1985) argued that this helps make healthier choices the easy choices. Tones and Tilford (1994) add that the goal of health promotion is the equable distribution of power and resources and this may involve challenging the impact on health of dominant ideologies such as the enterprise culture. Anderson (1983), writing for the WHO, concludes that three categories of health promotion activity emerge from these considerations. They are the action of individuals to improve health; interventions aimed at helping the preceding category be achieved; and those which act at a macro policy level and are thus independent of personal effort. For the WHO Jakarta Declaration (1997a) this means influencing the determinants of health so as to maximise health

---

BOX 1.4 DOMAINS OF HEALTH PROMOTION

- individual behaviour and lifestyle;
- social and environmental causes;
- health services.

(Tones 1990; Tones and Tilford 2001)

gain for people, reducing inequalities in health, furthering human rights and building social capital.

THE RELATIONSHIP BETWEEN HEALTH EDUCATION AND HEALTH PROMOTION

Although it is difficult to differentiate clearly between health education, disease prevention and health promotion a number of authors (Catford and Nutbeam 1984; Tones 1985; Tones and Tilford 2001; Whitehead 2004a) have endeavoured to clarify this relationship. The WHO (1986) contend that the area of overlap between health education and health promotion, as defined in the *Ottawa Charter*, is advocacy and supportive health policy. Tones (1985) similarly defines health promotion as the synthesis of health education and social engineering and for Tones (1993), Tones and Tilford (2001), Tones (2001) and Tones and Green (2004) health promotion is the sum of health education and healthy public policy.

Catford and Nutbeam (1984) define health education as information provision and advice on health risks and preventive behaviour via various media and the promotion of self-esteem and empowerment. They see health promotion as a means to improve and protect health through health education and personal services but also via biological, socio-economic and environmental interventions. It includes disease prevention and promoting positive health. Personal services comprise immunisation and screening, smoking cessation, keeping fit and weight control. Environmental interventions refer to more traditional public health measures such as sanitation, clean air, and health and safety regulations. Community development, organisational development and economic measures through fiscal policy, legislation and voluntary codes of practice are also placed under the heading of health promotion.

French (1985) contends that health promotion comprises health education as defined above plus curative medicine, legislative change and community development. Tannahill (1985) and Downie *et al.* (1990) argue that health promotion includes health education, prevention of disease and health protection. Health protection refers to disease and injury prevention and the promotion of positive health via legislation, policy, regulation and codes of conduct.

HEALTH EDUCATION, HEALTH PROMOTION AND NURSING

The debate in the nursing literature over the meaning of health education and health promotion, although far less extensive, is both informed by and is of the same tenor as the general debate. For example, Tomalin (1981), Brubaker (1983), Macleod Clark and Webb (1985), Latter *et al.* (1992), Macleod Clark *et al.* (1991), Delaney (1994), King (1994), Maben and Macleod Clark (1995), Norton (1998), Falk-Raphael (1999), Whitehead (2006) and Piper (2008) found confusion, ambiguity, vagueness and inconsistency over the meaning given to these concepts. Morgan and Marsh (1998) noted the narrow definition of health promotion emphasising individual risk factors, lifestyle and responsibility, i.e. orthodox disease prevention (Berg and Sarvimäki 2003). For Macleod Clark *et al.* (1996) health promotion was described in terms of lifestyle, behaviour change and thus contemporary definitions of health education. This attempt to clarify the meaning of health education and health promotion is accompanied by a lack of clarity over the knowledge and skills required by nurses to fulfil the role (Benson and Latter 1998) and the absence of a coherent health promotion strategy within acute settings (McBride 1994).

Tomalin (1981) found that, even within the variations of meaning, health education still constituted a narrow range of interventions. These ranged from telling patients how to take their medicines to collaborative nurse–patient interactions to determine patient needs and set shared and realistic goals. Consistent with a narrow focus, Macleod Clark and Webb (1985) aligned health education with patient teaching. The aim was to prepare patients intellectually and emotionally to make decisions on health-related matters. Such a limited approach explains how health promotion came to be seen as a process of communication in nursing and how this came to be the benchmark for measuring performance (Caraher 1994a). Hence, it evolved into a teaching rather than an educational experience reinforcing the inequality in power between the nurse and the patient. It also neglected to take account of social context and its influence on health-related behaviour (Caraher 1994a).

In a review of the American nursing literature Brubaker (1983) found common but superficial reference to health promotion. Few authors defined health promotion and there was a failure to differentiate between health promotion, disease prevention, health maintenance, community health and wellness and an inconsistency in their use. The interchangeable use of terms was also noted by Anderson (1984), Gott and O'Brien (1990a), Latter *et al.* (1992), King (1994) and Whitehead (2004a) but this is not the case for Parse (1990) who is adamant that prevention and health promotion are distinct. The former is a medical goal concerned with disease avoidance whereas health promotion involves measures to actively enhance the quality of life.

To complicate matters further, Pender (1996: 7) uses partially defined humanistic language to draw a distinction between health promotion and health protection but equates the latter with illness prevention. Pender outlines a number of distinguishing features. Health promotion is the underlying 'actualising tendency' that creates the motivation to change behaviour on the part of the individual and increase wellbeing, express 'human potential' and the 'quality of the flow of life in the human-environment interactive process'. Health promotion is not about specific disease, injury, or motivation to avoid these, whereas health protection/illness prevention, under-pinned by the 'stabilising tendency', is motivated by the desire and action for primary and secondary prevention of specific disease and injury and the preservation of homeostasis. Nevertheless, although distinct they are complementary and individual action may unite the two. For example, exercise may be taken for both positive and health protective reasons. Pender also acknowledges that social context is a major influence on health and can expand or inhibit human potential and wellbeing and that nurses should work to address inequality. More contentiously she advocates that nurses should role-model healthy lifestyles.

Brubaker (1983), however, contends that health promotion is neither synonymous with any of the terms used interchangeably by others nor with rehabilitation; the latter accords with Anderson (1984) and many nursing commentators who also distinguish health promotion from care and rehabilitation (Delaney 1994). The themes that emerged from Brubaker's (1983) review of the literature suggest that positive health is also more than health maintenance and disease prevention. Health promotion is health education as defined in the previous section (including self-development and personal growth) and social engineering. Inherent features are disease prevention, health mainten-ance and stability, but these are not the primary focus as they merely seek to preserve the status quo.

King (1994) also contends that health promotion has a broad focus beyond disease prevention and health maintenance to preserve homeostasis and is concerned with improving health in terms of personal growth, wellness (physical, mental and social wellbeing) and quality of life. King (1994) talks of involving people in a participatory capacity, of devolving control and of the goal of positive health and wellbeing, but these concepts are not defined. This is in part because King sees the latter two as qualitative in nature. The meaning of a wellness approach to intervention is also unclear. What is evident is that health promotion is a politically oriented multi-sectoral activity that embraces social, economic and ecological objectives alongside those of an individual behavioural nature.

While Lask (1987) broadens the definition of health education to include social and environmental elements in line with the early definitions in the general literature, Latter *et al.* (1992) see the role here for health education as raising public awareness about these issues. For Latter (1998), health education is a feature of a broad and highly inclusive definition of health promotion that also embraces advocacy, public policy, legislation and community development. From a nursing perspective, however, Latter (2001) contends that hospital nurses' contribution to health promotion is mostly, although not exclusively, within the realm of health education and at the level of nurse–patient interaction. For Latter (2001), much of the emphasis has been on helping patients understand the disease process and its management and helping them understand and prepare for procedures such as surgery. Latter (2001) also highlights that, while often concerned with compliance and didactic approaches, such interventions are known to have a beneficial effect by reducing anxiety and accelerating recovery.

Latter *et al.* (1992) include empowerment, which focuses on partnership and fostering patient self-esteem and self-efficacy, within their definition of health education. Other authors in the nursing literature also emphasise empowerment as part of health education (Lask 1987) but some go further in advancing it as a part of health education within health promotion (Tones 1993) and as a part of health promotion (Wilson-Barnett and Latter 1993). Indeed Tones (2001) contends that a key issue is the extent to which health care professionals operationalise the empowerment part of their health promotion role. Thus Latter *et al.* (1992) conclude that health education is the preferable descriptor to health promotion.

Caraher (1994a) opts for the term health promotion and adopts Nutbeam's (1986) definition. Health promotion is a broader concept than health education and Caraher maintains that it can embrace the role of the nurse as patient advocate. This view is shared by Minkler (1989), who aligns it with education as a process of nurturing and enabling. Caraher (1994a) then contradicts this by suggesting that the hospital setting in both demanding compliance and order and the professionalisation of nursing militates against patient involvement and autonomy, and thus health promotion.

Green and Raeburn (1988) also champion the advocate, mediator and supporter aspects of the health promotion role of health professionals, and Dines and Cribb (1993) refer to health promotion as an advocacy of certain values in line with the WHO principles of health promotion. The role of the nurse in relation to the latter is to be aware of the impact practice and policies have on health, and help to put health on the agenda of policy makers. But the central question for Dines and Cribb (1993) that should constantly be posed is not what are the domains of health promotion, but is health promotion being done in a health promoting way? From the point of view of health promotion and the health service this seems to translate into reorienting it in a manner compatible with the WHO values (Dines and Cribb 1993).

Caraher (1994a), Delaney (1994), King (1994), Maben and Macleod Clark (1995) and Norton (1998) conclude that health promotion is an inclusive umbrella phrase or overarching concept (Wilson-Barnett and Latter 1993; Latter 1998) that denotes competing philosophies and approaches. As an overarching concept, it can provide a philosophical guide to practice that should coincide with other nursing goals and reflect an awareness of the range of influences on health. This can translate into encouraging consumerism and participation to create a flexible, collaborative and a more personal service based on patient-defined needs, choice, independence and free will and thus an acknowledgement of a plurality of values and ways of living (Wilson-Barnett and Latter 1993). It would reject inequality of service provision, although quite how resources are to be distributed more fairly in relation to the above is not made entirely clear by Wilson-Barnett and Latter (1993).

27

THE MEANING OF HEALTH PROMOTION: OPERATIONAL DEFINITION

Despite the plethora of contested meanings, for the purpose of this book it would seem fair to conclude that health education is a key element of, but not synonymous with, health promotion (Tones and Tilford 2001; Tones and Green 2004). Health education and health promotion are distinct but interlinked, with the latter having active involvement of an informed public and the former as a critical tool to achieve this outcome (Nutbeam 1986). Although each contains subordinate themes, broadly speaking health education is concerned with both top-down and bottom-up individual action perspectives. Health promotion incorporates health education and legislative, public health and social policy, political and communitarian interventions.

Anderson (1983) encapsulates the general debate and defines health promotion as health education combined with socio-political/economic intervention for behaviour and environmental change, health protection and improvement.

Although dated and not the most fluid or succinct of definitions, from a specific nursing perspective Maben and Macleod Clark (1995: 1163) offer their inclusive and more detailed thoughts on health promotion, which dovetail with the above:

> Health promotion is an attempt to improve the health status of an individual or community, and is also concerned with the prevention of disease, though this is not its only purpose, as health is not merely the absence of disease. At its broadest level it is concerned with the wider influences on health and therefore with the policy and legislative imperative of these. Health education through information giving, advice, support and skills training is part of, and a necessary prerequisite to, health promotion, attempts to raise awareness of the issues in question and fosters an ability to cope with illness or disease. More radically, health promotion is in itself an approach to care through empowerment, equity, collaboration and participation, and may involve social and environmental change.

Thus, put succinctly but with a more contemporary spin, health education in nursing is concerned with health/illness-related information, learning and behaviour change whereas health promotion is concerned with a socio-political policy agenda, community health in general and community empowerment in particular (Whitehead 2004a). In addition, and consistent with Tones and Green (2004), primary, secondary and tertiary health promotion are defined in Box 1.5 together with quaternary health promotion (Scriven 2005).

HEALTH PROMOTION AND NURSE EDUCATION

Much of the literature aligns health promotion in nursing with traditional perspectives (Whitehead 2003, 2006) and narrow forms of intervention. Practice has not been associated with the range of activities identified by the *Ottawa Charter* (WHO 1986), the mainstream literature or modern public health nursing (DoH 2003). Whitehead (2003, 2006) and Piper (2008) contend that nurses are failing to conceptualise the difference between health education and health promotion and adopt contemporary meanings. In his comprehensive review of health promotion and nursing education, Whitehead

BOX 1.5 PRIMARY, SECONDARY AND TERTIARY HEALTH PROMOTION; QUATERNARY HEALTH PROMOTION

- Primary health promotion refers to interventions to prevent new cases of disease or injury. It is concerned with asymptomatic disease detection (Tones 1981) and 'stopping ill health arising in the first place' (Orme et al. 2007: 342). Tones (1997) refers to primary prevention as health behaviour.
- Secondary health promotion aims to minimise the consequences of disease or injury, prevent them from becoming chronic or irreversible and to restore the patient to their former health status. Secondary prevention is illness behaviour (Tones 1997) and includes using the appropriate health services as and when needed (Tones 1981).
- Tertiary health promotion aims to maximise health experience within the constraints imposed by a chronic disease (for example, diabetes, asthma, HIV), injury or concomitant disability, prevent restrictions or further complications and to assist rehabilitation. Both secondary and tertiary health promotion are concerned with disease-related behaviour. Tones (1997) refers to tertiary prevention as the sick role and together primary, secondary and tertiary prevention constitute the sickness career (Tones 1997 is drawing on the work of Kasl and Cobb 1966)
- Quaternary health promotion (Scriven 2005) seeks to promote bio-psycho-social health in the terminal phase of disease.

(Tones and Green 2004; and Scriven 2005)

(2007a) highlights that this is reflected in outdated nurse education curricula with its medical model approach mistakenly aligned with health promotion, not just historically but in current practice.

The concern is that if mainstream language is not being used to teach nursing students, then the nursing voice may not be heard by other disciplines (Gottlieb 1992) and may become 'invisible' (Falk-Rafael 1999, cited in Whitehead 2006). This may result in nursing failing to make a full contribution to the health promotion theory and practice debate. The reorientation of UK health policy over the last decade (DoH 1992, 1993, 1999a, 1999b, 2000) emphasising health promotion as a health service priority and placing it explicitly on the nursing agenda makes this more significant than ever.

Thus, while there is no one final, incontestable definition of health promotion (Whitehead 2004a), nurse educators need to at least offer definitions of health promotion for nursing (Berg and Sarvimäki 2003) and nursing practice (Robinson and Hill 1998) couched in the language of health policy and of other disciplines to facilitate both understanding and a contribution to the wider debate. Using and making explicit contemporary language and its meaning also has to be embedded in the nursing curriculum and associated teaching and learning strategies for the twenty-first century.

If nursing wants to make a full contribution to health promotion the philosophy and organisational structures underpinning practice (Robinson and Hill 1998; Northrup and Purkis 2001) must also be clearly articulated and this needs to be a feature of concomitant curricula (Rush 1997). This should be accompanied by a clear outline of the aims, methods and outcomes of the various models of health education/health promotion and their strengths and weaknesses to contextualise the terminology in relation to practice (Piper 2008). Such an approach would be consistent with Whitehead's (2003) call for nurses to adopt a structured and systematic approach to health promotion.

Although it remains important to focus on the traditional and 'visible' (Rush 1997) aspects of health promotion and to utilise different teaching strategies to facilitate learning about these (Hsiao *et al.* 2005), socio-political factors such as inequalities (the less visible) must also be addressed (Morgan and Marsh 1998; Robinson and Hill 1998; Burke and Smith 2000). Hence, Whitehead (2004a, 2006) contends that socio-political approaches such as community development have superseded individualistic forms of health promotion, and nursing (and thus nurse education) should attempt to reflect this wider agenda. This may also require alternative models of teaching (Falk-Rafael *et al.* 2004) and stronger engagement with public health concepts, models and theory.

PUBLIC HEALTH, HEALTH DEVELOPMENT AND HEALTH IMPROVEMENT

The first point of reference for the WHO (1998a) when defining public health is the Acheson (1988) report into public health in the UK. Acheson defines it as organised interventions using art and science for:

- disease prevention
- promoting health
- extending life.

The report highlights the narrow definition given to the term public health historically and how it came to be associated with health improvement via sanitation, communicable disease management and related epidemiological surveillance at the expense of lifestyle influences. Acheson (1988) emphasised that the latter was equally important in promoting health and that any conceptual gap between preventive and curative medicine is a false dichotomy.

For Acheson (1988), public health includes both preventing or minimising the negative impact on health of environmental, social and behavioural influences and the provision of good quality health care for those in need, including dentistry, pharmacy, etc. The report acknowledges that health is influenced by socio-economic factors including housing, employment and poverty and that the promotion of health involves all elements of society. It requires not only the effective co-ordination of national policy across UK government departments (i.e. not just the Department of Health), the local policy of health authorities, local authorities and the voluntary sector but should also involve industry, the media and the action of individuals in preserving their own health.

The WHO (1998a) shares this socio-political view of public health and, together with Naidoo and Wills (2005), see it as an all-embracing or umbrella concept that subsumes health promotion. The WHO (1998a) also acknowledge the concept of the 'new' public health alluded to by Acheson (1988) which is concerned to take account of the impact of lifestyle and social context on health and develop strategies for fostering healthy lifestyles (focus on individual) and supportive environments (focus on communities). Although Baggott (2000) acknowledges that public health is a broad church he (Baggott 2004) contends that there is a consensus over its primary focus on collective health improvement rather than disease management in individuals. Orme et al. (2007) also stress the population perspective in their definition of public health, which is otherwise in line with Acheson (1988) above.

This clarity of definition is slightly muddied by the additional term health development. The WHO (1998a) define this as the progressive and continuous health gain of individuals and communities, with the Jakarta Declaration (WHO 1997a) referring to health promotion as a pivotal component of health development with the five priorities for the twenty-first century of:

- promoting social responsibility for health;
- increasing investments for health development;

- consolidating and expanding partnerships for health;
- increasing community capacity and empowering the individual;
- securing an infrastructure for health promotion.

The WHO (1985) *Targets for Health for All* European regional strategy outlines lifestyles and health; risk factors; and reorientation of health services as the main areas for health development. To achieve health improvement in these areas requires political, organisational, technological and research activity to achieve the four major aims in Box 1.6.

The WHO Jakarta Declaration (1997a) calls for the use of a range of approaches for effective health development and states that a combination of the five strategies of the *Ottawa Charter*, i.e. the core elements of health promotion, are the way to achieve this throughout the world. The challenge is to find ways to catalyse health promotion and develop partnerships for health and social development across the various sectors of society and within local communities and families.

It is then, quite difficult to differentiate between health promotion and health development but seemingly the former helps achieve the latter and thus health improvement. However, as Earle (2007) points out, definitions and meanings given to concepts change over time and in practice some of these terms are used interchangeably. What is important to internalise here is that whatever descriptor is used all forms of nursing involve the promotion of health and, as the Jakarta Declaration (WHO 1997a) states, there is clear evidence that:

- a settings approach offers practical opportunities for the implementation of the strategies, for example communities, schools, the workplace and health care facilities;

BOX 1.6 THE FOUR MAJOR AIMS OF HEALTH IMPROVEMENT

- 'Equity in health between and within countries';
  and adding:
- 'life to years';
- 'health to life';
- 'years to life'.

(WHO 1985: 9; WHO 1991c: 5)

- public participation with people involved in the decision-making process is central to health promotion success;
- access to education and information for health learning is essential to achieve the above and for individual and community empowerment.

All of the above fit on the spectrum of nursing with nurses as pivotal figures working with individuals, communities, environments and nations to improve health. Thus, the WHO Munich Declaration (2000) and the RCN (2007) believe that nurses have a crucial part to play in contributing to public health via health promotion by influencing health policy and by helping to:

- positively influence health-related behaviour for a longer life;
- reduce inequalities in health;
- improve the health of populations;
- facilitate the development of social capital;
- reorientate health services.

CONCLUSION

Health, health education, health promotion and public health are all contested concepts, i.e. their definition and meaning has been debated and disputed. This chapter has sought to provide an overview of the conceptual wrangling and arrive at a point of consensus for nursing consistent with the general literature and health policy. It is important to note here then, that for the purpose of this book health education is top-down health-related behaviour (the nurse as behaviour change agent) and bottom-up empowerment (the nurse as empowerment facilitator) individual action interventions that are part of health promotion. However, the latter also includes top-down strategic/ policy (the nurse as strategic practitioner) and bottom-up collective empowerment interventions, but is itself subsumed within public health. The point is that as Gottlieb (1992) contends, careful use of language is crucial for describing and evaluating nursing approaches to health promotion. Crucial because if nursing wants to make a meaningful contribution it must reflect mainstream terminology or it will not be heard by other disciplines and thus will be disadvantaged when trying to influence an important contemporary debate and associated policy and practice issues.

LEARNING TRIGGERS

Having read Chapter 1, complete the learning triggers below to reinforce your critical understanding of the concepts that have been discussed:

- Define health.
- Summarise the relationship between disease and illness.
- Define health education, health promotion and summarise the relationship between them.
- Summarise the relationship between health education, health promotion and nursing.
- Define primary, secondary and tertiary health promotion.
- Define public health, health development and health improvement.

OPERATIONAL DEFINITIONS AND THEORY-TESTING CRITERIA

2

INTRODUCTION

The purpose of this chapter is to comply with Rawson's (2002) call for a debate between health promotion frameworks and their philosophical foundations rather than continuing to focus on models within frameworks. It is also concerned to identify and apply criteria for appraising health promotion frameworks to help establish what makes a theoretically robust structure. It does these tasks in the following ways. In borrowing from Piper's (2004) unpublished qualitative theory-testing research it first, identifies appropriate delineating terminology, defines what constitutes a framework of health promotion and establishes the relationship between these and theories and models. Second, the quality assessment criteria (Greener and Grimshaw 1996), which are used to judge and compare their theoretical rigour, breadth and depth, are outlined. The criteria are for establishing how a health promotion framework can be internally validated as a benchmark by which to measure others, i.e. to develop, synthesise and validate the framework of the book as a tool for operational use by nurses and to gauge its 'fitness for practice' and the credentials of competing frameworks.

Finally, Chapter 2 summarises and applies the theory-testing criteria to evaluate and gauge the robustness of Beattie's (1991) general health promotion framework from which the nursing health promotion frameworks of Piper and Brown (1998a), Piper (2000, 2004, 2007a, 2007b) and the framework of the book derive. This process includes juxtaposing Beattie's (1991) work with structurally compatible frameworks and those with explicit socio-political elements for comparative analysis. In addition, the complementary theoretical structures of health and cultural bias are introduced to contextualise further, in terms of socio-political philosophy, the models of health promotion within the framework and augment its analytical properties.

FRAMEWORKS

Frameworks of health promotion are described by a number of authors who use various terms such as schema, structural map, typology, etc. This potential for ambiguity and conceptual confusion has been avoided herein through use of the term framework, which, for the purpose of clarity and consistency, supplants any other term used to describe a theoretical structure that classifies models of health education and health promotion.

Frameworks are like taxonomies in that they identify, name, describe, group and classify phenomena into ordered categories and communicate the nature, limits and realm of a discipline (Bircher 1975). In classifying and organising concepts they also illustrate the relationship between them (Polit and Beck 2006) and, in charting and guiding knowledge already plotted, should be thought of metaphorically like geographical maps (Visintainer 1986). Taxonomies broadly outline the focus of enquiry of a discipline (Adam 1985), the founding knowledge that guides research decisions (Fawcett 1991), and organise phenomena that are linked by their relationship to a common theme (Polit and Hungler 1993).

Rather than used in a hierarchical manner, which Suppe and Jacox (1985) usually associate with taxonomies, the term is used herein as described by Rawson and Grigg (1988). They describe taxonomy as a non-hierarchical system of classification and contrast it with typology, which they see as a dimensional or hierarchical framework with graded distinctions between models. As structures that integrate abstract and general concepts into meaningful configuration, taxonomies and thus frameworks serve as a tool to evaluate the adequacy of theories (Suppe and Jacox 1985).

THEORY DEFINITION AND THE RELATIONSHIP BETWEEN THEORY AND TAXONOMIES (FRAMEWORKS)

Based on a general summation of the views of a number of authors (Kerlinger 1964; Ellis 1968; Schutz 1971; Laudan 1981; Turner 1987; Marriner-Tomey 1989; Rawson 2002; Polit and Beck 2006), theories can be defined in the following way. Theories specify relationships and the connections between, and organise or integrate collections of propositions, concepts and variables. They refine levels of understanding, create a general frame of reference and hold fundamental views about social phenomena and an immutable commitment to a world-view. Theories explain and predict phenomena and explain empirical data that can then be tested against the facts and make findings meaningful.

While the above definition is helpful, it is insufficient for the purpose of this study as it makes no reference to the relationship between a theory and a taxonomy (i.e. framework) or to levels of theorising. Interested in the role of theory in the practice discipline of nursing, Dickoff *et al.* (1968) see theories as conceptual frameworks or (Dickoff and James 1968) as devices or systems invented with the ultimate goal of producing desired change in the nursing situation and in the patient (Meleis 1985). Dickoff *et al.* (1968) group theories into the four hierarchical levels specified below, with the higher and more complex categories building on the lower categories:

- factor-isolating theories;
- factor-relating theories;
- situation-relating theories;
- situation-producing theories.

At the simplest and thus foundation theory level, factor-isolating theories identify, label, name and introduce technical terminology, classify and categorise concepts and may appear quite primitive. After isolated concepts have been named, described and classified, factor-relating theories depict and propose rather than test relationships and correlations between concepts and phenomena. The factor-relating level provides a robust descriptive theoretical base for nursing (Morse and Field 1985).

Situation-relating theory is of a lower order causal-connection and predictive nature. Situation-producing or fourth-level (Dickoff and James 1968) theory, the pinnacle of theory development, is practice theory of an advanced predictive nature and enables the manipulation of variables and phenomena to produce the desired nursing outcomes of a situation. As can be seen from the above definitions, a health promotion framework (taxonomy) is a form of theory, albeit a lower order factor-isolating and/or factor-relating theory, and is the bedrock of, and a prerequisite for subsequent and more advanced (situation-relating/producing) theory.

MODELS

Given that it is health promotion models that are classified in the literature by the frameworks (taxonomies) it is important to draw a distinction between these and theory. A model represents reality and the key aspects of a subject area in a simplified but meaningful way (Tones and Tilford 2001). They are not necessary components of theory building but help make theory concrete (Rawson 2002). They provide essential analogies and mental imagery to grasp theoretical entities, help thinking unfold and act as a form of intellectual scaffolding to support concept building (Fallding 1971). From a nursing perspective, models in general help with the perception of illness and nursing needs of patients in a particular way. They influence how nurses understand and interpret disease, how related needs and appropriate nursing care is identified to meet those needs and how the interventions should be evaluated (Cormack and Reynolds 1992).

Rawson and Grigg (1988) and Rawson (1990) distinguish between iconic and analogic models. Applied to health promotion, iconic models are pragmatic and simplified descriptions of practice low on the scale of theoretical complexity and abstraction. Analogic models are abstract metaphorical explanatory systems designed to aid conceptual understanding of the relationship between elements of the model and may lack practical application.

Further distinction and clarification is offered by Tones and Tilford (2001) who differentiate between ideological models and technical models. Ideological models precede technical models in that they are foundation constructions that guide health promotion practice and outline the strategic purpose of intervention. They are based on a system of beliefs, values and philosophy. Technical models go further and help to translate ideological commitments into a more systematic and organised form of intervention based on a comprehensive understanding, interpretation and explanation of social phenomena and means of evaluating practice. The focus of this book is on both; i.e. lower order factor-isolating/relating theory as a way of classifying models of health promotion in an ideological way and on the technical as described above in relation to pragmatic nursing practice.

CRITERIA FOR TESTING THE CONCEPTUAL ADEQUACY OF HEALTH PROMOTION FRAMEWORKS (TAXONOMIES)

The critique of commonly used concepts requires the creation of a measuring stick against which they can be measured, examined and compared (Feyerbend 1975). In terms of health promotion, the scarcity of literature on how to develop conceptual models for research and practice (Earp and Ennett 1991) is equalled by the dearth of published work on what constitutes a robust framework. A notable exception to this are Kerlinger's (1964) rules of categorisation. Although these were developed as part of a guide on the principles of analysis and interpretation of data from behavioural research, there is no reason to suggest that they cannot be used as a framework for other systems of classification (Bircher 1975).

Scrutiny of Kerlinger's (1964) original work reveals that Bircher (1975) has interpreted and translated the categories for taxonomy development that she has applied to the concept of nursing diagnosis. It is a slightly modified version of her work that is used herein and outlined in Box 2.1 as foundation criteria for judging the adequacy of health promotion frameworks. These can be strengthened by adding modified elements of Fawcett's (1995) criteria for evaluating conceptual frameworks of nursing as shown in Box 2.2.

Although there is some overlap with criteria already identified, the application of some of that more usually reserved for ascertaining the conceptual adequacy of theories can be utilised to assist further in determining the conceptual adequacy of health promotion frameworks. When judging what makes theory productive and useful, an understanding of its characteristics beyond simple definitions and an

**BOX 2.1 FIVE CATEGORIES FOR HEALTH PROMOTION
FRAMEWORK DEVELOPMENT**

- The framework is relevant to the purpose or research problem and each category reflects one view of the world.
- The framework is exhaustive: all possible items can be coded into one or other of the categories of the system.
- Individual categories of the framework are clearly defined and mutually exclusive: a given item can be placed in only one category of the set.
- The framework is derived from and fully develops a principle of ordering.
- The categories of the framework are on the same level of discourse or abstraction.

(after Bircher 1975)

**BOX 2.2 CRITERIA FOR EVALUATING CONCEPTUAL FRAMEWORKS
IN NURSING**

- Explication of origins: the philosophical premise of the framework is made explicit; the theorists who influenced the author of the framework are acknowledged.
- Comprehensiveness of content: the framework provides adequate breadth and depth in its description of categories.
- Logical congruence: the internal structure of the framework is logically congruent; the framework reflects logical reformulation and translation of diverse perspectives.
- Credibility and social utility: the framework can be used to guide practice.

(after Fawcett 1995)

evaluation of the extent to which it provides a robust explanation and interpretation of social reality is required (Judd *et al.* 1991). A number of authors have identified criteria for testing the plausibility of theory and these are summarised in Box 2.3. A good, i.e. a theoretically sound, health promotion framework would meet the combined requirements of the criteria of Bircher (1975), Fawcett (1995) and the other authors referred to in Box 2.3.

BOX 2.3 CRITERIA FOR DETERMINING THEORETICAL PLAUSIBILITY

- Internal consistency (Campbell 1981; Suppe and Jacox 1985; Judd *et al*. 1991): no internal inconsistencies or contradictions and compatible and mutually supporting assumptions (Campbell 1981).
- Coherence, comprehensibility and accessibility (Judd *et al*. 1991).
- Conceptual adequacy and logical development (Suppe and Jacox 1985).
- Simplicity (Suppe and Jacox 1985; Marriner-Tomey 1989): comprehensive, concrete, understandable theory with strong conceptual inter-relationships (Marriner-Tomey 1989).
- Clarity: precise definition of key terms with central contentions and assumptions clearly stated and congruent (Campbell 1981; Marriner-Tomey 1989).
- Explanatory adequacy (Campbell 1981).
- Generality: the scope, breadth, depth and complexity of concepts (Marriner-Tomey 1989).
- Derivable consequences: the ability to guide and validate research practice (Marriner-Tomey 1989).
- Scope: frames and integrates a broad number of concepts with its force directly related to its breadth (Ellis 1968).
- Clinical usefulness: its ability to guide nursing practice which, for Ellis (1968), is the key and ultimate test of significance.

41

HEALTH PROMOTION FRAMEWORK EXEMPLAR

To help nurses make a judgement about the practical and clinical worth of a model (or in this case a framework of models) Cormack and Reynolds (1992) contend that it is important that nurses are fully informed about its origins and the extent to which the work derives from tested and established theory. They add that models should be developed from theory with scientific integrity and that for nurses to make full use of a model there must be clarity of thought and language and that it should have been subjected to theory testing.

In addition, when writing on the professional ideology of social pathologists in relation to the sociology of knowledge, Mills (1943) expressed his concern about the lack of theoretical abstraction and the theoretical weakness of this group of social scientists. He took the view that simple evaluations will be perpetuated in the absence of a construction and an understanding of total social structures. The literature reveals that charges of this type could also be levelled at a considerable number of health promotion theorists.

A notable exception to the charge of Mills is the work of Beattie (1991), modified for nursing by Piper and Brown (1998a), and Piper (2000, 2004, 2007a, 2007b), who is critical of the paucity of systematic analysis and academic scrutiny of the work of his contemporaries. He contends that his framework of models of health promotion has been subject to rigorous academic scrutiny based on sociological insight.

Beattie (1993) also applies this type of analysis and synthesis to the concept of health. In a repeat of his 1991 design he constructs a distinct but complementary framework of models of health with compatible philosophical, socio-political and socio-cultural outcomes. While the latter, augmented by the grid/group analysis of Douglas (1982), was most helpful as an analytical tool for theory development and synthesis, for Rawson and Grigg (1988) Beattie's health promotion structural map stands alone as the only truly analogic, purpose built framework of integrated health promotion models. This in part explains why it was selected as the exemplar herein, i.e. the theory base for deriving a health-promotion nursing framework.

A second reason for selecting Beattie's (1991) health promotion framework is that it facilitates the analysis of authoritative and emancipatory power structures. It helps illustrate the ownership of knowledge (Rawson and Grigg 1988), issues of power and control in the client–practitioner relationship (Naidoo and Wills 2000) and delineates individual and collective modes of intervention. It makes these points of convergence and divergence and the tensions and conflicts between them explicit and helps clarify the options that are enabled by the competing models.

Beattie's framework highlights both clear strategies for health promotion intervention and that each model is based on a political and social policy philosophy. It also depicts the relationship between models and goes beyond the classifying and categorising factor-isolating theory to the factor-relating theory category (Dickoff et al. 1968). In going beyond simple description, his work illustrates and enables an assessment of the founding ideological and epistemological (metatheoretical) origins of models of health promotion, health and cultural bias and the polarities, norms and assumptions that underpin them.

Beattie's (1991) framework comprises the four distinct, and for Beattie mutually exclusive, health promotion models of health persuasion techniques; personal counselling for health; legislative action for health; and community development for health. They emerge when the authoritative/negotiated (mode of intervention) and individual/collective (focus of intervention) bi-polar dimensions, which derive from long-standing, enduring and unresolved social theory conflicts and multiple sources, are intersected to create his 'structural map', illustrated in Figure 2.1.

The models of health promotion represent clusters of theories and interventions and thus a framework of ideological (Tones and Tilford 2001) or analogic (Rawson and Grigg 1988; Rawson 1990) models of health promotion. Each of these models creates a different relationship between the health promoter and the public due to different aims, methods and outcomes of intervention. Their juxtaposition highlights also their convergent and divergent philosophical positions. Rawson and Grigg (1988) revised and reorientated an earlier version of Beattie's health promotion taxonomy to depict the four approaches as truly discrete, i.e. mutually exclusive, entities. They considered this to be more consistent with his use of the concepts and distinct stance of his models.

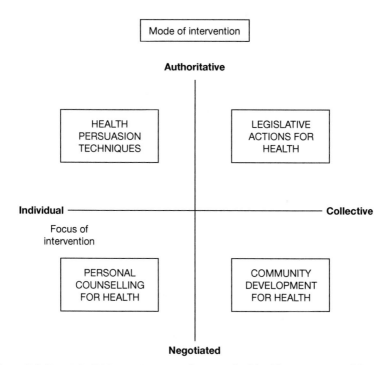

Figure 2.1 Beattie's (1991: 167, Fig 7.1) framework of health promotion models

Health persuasion techniques and personal counselling for health are united by their individual focus of intervention as both are concerned with various aspects of personal behaviour and lifestyle, but are polarised by the rival positions they occupy on the mode of intervention dimension. The latter is essentially an indicator of power and control and beliefs about social order and epistemology. It is where health persuasion techniques align with legislative action for health, and personal counselling for health with community development for health. Legislative action for health, and community development for health come together on the collective side of the focus of intervention dimensions where health promotion is about structural issues, policy development and community action and community empowerment issues respectively.

The top-down, expert-led health persuasion techniques derives its power base from traditional, objective, scientific and medical research on the relationship between diseases such as coronary heart disease, risk factors and lifestyle. This information-based model simplifies and disseminates research outcomes via a range of mass media (TV, newspapers, magazines, posters, leaflets, etc.) health campaigns and via health care professionals. The need for bodily regulation and the controlling and correcting of attitudinal and behavioural inadequacies in individuals are emphasised, together with the risks and dangers to them if they fail to pursue the prescribed course of action.

Personal counselling for health is a bottom-up client-centred personal development and empowerment approach rooted in humanistic psychology. The focus is on individual life-review, reflection and clarification on the scope for personal life change and self-determination based on the subjective perceptions and life-choices of the client. Health promotion interventions are grounded in process and may entail social- and life-skills training to build confidence and self-esteem, develop assertiveness, decision-making and action-planning skills. Outcomes, for example with young people, might be the ability to resist unwanted social pressure. Its holistic stance further differentiates personal counselling for health from health persuasion techniques as the latter tends to focus on a particular topic at any one time, such as coronary heart disease, HIV/AIDS or smoking.

Legislative action for health is a top-down cluster of interventions. Collective health is improved through enacting health, welfare and economic legislation and by implementing policy decisions to address health determinants and social inequalities. The historical roots of this approach lay in the late nineteenth and early twentieth century environmental and public health interventions that introduced clean water, sanitation and better housing.

This approach has also come to embrace food and agricultural policies and taxation of harmful substances such as cigarettes. More contemporary developments and offshoots of legislative action for health include the UK Healthy Cities Project, food and health policies at the devolved level of Health and Local Education Authorities and change at an institutional level (for example, hospitals, schools and the workplace).

As with the legislative action for health, community development for health is collective in its focus of intervention but its mode of intervention is bottom-up. It operates from a community action and collective empowerment stance with the power and impetus for action stemming from members of the community. Similarly, social factors are seen as the major influence on health rather than individual health-related behaviours, disease prevention or issues of personal control, autonomy and self-esteem.

Community development for health is where groups of like-minded people with shared problems come together to articulate their concerns and to construct a mutually agreed agenda for social and micro-structural change. This is based explicitly on their subjective perceptions of problems and expressed needs and is mostly related to the physical and social environment within which they live. It is a collective empowerment approach where otherwise powerless and alienated individuals find a voice through uniting forces. The facilitative role of the health promoter is to help identify and bring together groups of people with shared concerns, to fulfil the 'gate-keeper' role by helping groups gain access to power holders, to assist with networking and help mobilise resources for local change. Examples might include, improvement to the physical environment, access to services or developments such as safe play areas for children.

INTERNAL THEORY TESTING OF BEATTIE'S (1991) HEALTH PROMOTION FRAMEWORK

In order to verify theoretically Beattie's (1991) work as the benchmark health promotion framework for testing the merit of others, its theoretical rigour and adequacy are internally tested against the criteria advanced by Bircher (1975) (see Box 2.1), Fawcett (1995) (see Box 2.2) and the accompanying indicators of theoretical plausibility. In terms of Bircher's criteria, Beattie's framework reflects opposing world-views of health promotion and is relevant for the purpose of this book. The framework can account comprehensively (although perhaps not exhaustively) for the conceptual constructions advanced by other authors, and allows for them to be coded with varying degrees of fit into one of the four models. Individual models are clearly defined and described on the same level of abstraction and are mutually exclusive in that interventions are specific to one of the models.

Beattie's (1991) framework conforms to Bircher's (1975) criteria of deriving from and fully developing a principle of ordering and to Fawcett's (1995) explication of origins. The latter requires the philosophical premise to be made explicit and the theorists who influenced the author of the framework to be acknowledged. The framework is also consistent with Fawcett's other criteria. The content is comprehensive and provides adequate depth and breadth in its description of categories. Its internal structure is logically congruent in its cross-classification and translation of diverse perspectives. It has high credibility and social utility in that it can be used to guide health promotion strategic thinking, planning and practice.

Beattie's health promotion framework also offers theoretical plausibility. There are no internal inconsistencies or contradictions and assumptions are compatible and mutually supporting. It offers coherence, clarity, comprehensibility, conceptual adequacy and logical development with clear statements about central contentions. It has explanatory adequacy and depth and it answers the call of Ellis (1968) for scope in being able to frame and integrate a broad number of concepts. Most importantly, Beattie's framework passes the ultimate test of significance; its potential to guide planning and practice means that it has clinical usefulness. Indeed Rawson (2002) contends that it influenced at least one era of health education. In addition, the framework meets with Guba and Lincoln's (1989) call for its ability to accommodate new information and new levels of sophistication as they emerge.

Constructive criticism of Beattie's (1991) health promotion framework

For Mills (1959), good classification of theory requires the criteria to be made explicit and this is best achieved by cross-classification, by considering extremes and polarised ideas that will help identify the dimensions of the debate and elucidate meaning from the relationship between contrasting perspectives. Beattie (1991) contends that his framework adopts the cross-classification device of Mills (1959) to enumerate his four models of health promotion. The framework, and variations on the theme, which are aligned to wider theoretical frameworks by Beattie is, however, based on interpretation and extrapolation of the ideas of Mills (1959) as no diagrammatic device appears in the work of the latter referred to in the chapter.

Similar analytical frameworks of social theory have also been developed by Burrell and Morgan (1979) and Robertson (1974) and applied as operational health promotion framework by others (Caplan and Holland 1990; Taylor 1990) writing at a similar time to Beattie (1991), although he makes no mention of their work. In addition, Jones and Naidoo (2000) highlight the problem created for practitioners by the Beattie health promotion framework if their interventions do not fit neatly into one of the models but embrace different approaches.

FRAMEWORKS OF HEALTH (BEATTIE 1993) AND CULTURAL BIAS (DOUGLAS 1982)

This book concurs with the views of Jones and Naidoo (2000) and Naidoo and Wills (2000) that Beattie's (1991) health promotion framework can serve well as an effective tool for identifying and examining the assumptions that underpin practice. For Jones and Naidoo (2000), the latter is merely the empirical manifestation of fundamental social ideologies and conflicts. This level of analysis, making explicit the links between models of health promotion and their philosophical foundations referred to by Jones and Naidoo (2000), is also developed in relation to health by Beattie (1993) and cultural bias via reference to the grid/group analysis of Douglas (1982).

Naidoo and Wills (2000) highlight the conceptual relationship between the models in Beattie's 1991 and 1993 frameworks. Although offering a continuity of format and many of the virtues of the earlier work, the focus on health by Beattie (1993) means that it is unsuitable as a stand-alone framework of choice for this book on health promotion. This argument also applies to the framework of cultural bias of Douglas (1982). However, as complementary conceptual devices, they are outlined here to demonstrate the alignment of their inherent models with Beattie's 1991 work and as additional frameworks for the synthesis and contextualisation of the framework of the book. They are then deployed in this book in the true sense of the framework as defined earlier. In line with Beattie (1991, 1993), Jones and Naidoo (2000) and Naidoo and Wills (2000), they are used as a basis for classifying competing theoretical and empirical health promotion positions and general areas of demarcation.

In addition, the assertion of these authors that there is a conceptual fit between the Beattie 1991 and 1993 frameworks, and the contention by Beattie (1993) of the relationship between the framework of health and cultural bias, are accepted. Thus, detailed analysis of any potential subtle difference or conflict between, for example, the communitarian model of health and community development for health and where the former might see limits to community empowerment if this were at the expense of individual empowerment are not a feature of the discussion.

Beattie's (1991) framework illustrates and clarifies the conflicting and dichotomous models of contemporary health promotion and their political philosophies and orientations. In line with this, Beattie's (1993) framework pursues a similar but distinctive process. It moves the debate from health promotion to the relationship between competing health beliefs and narratives in contemporary society and discrete socio-political views of the social world in relation to his earlier (1991) structure. Beattie (1993) also outlines the socio-cultural perspective of the models of health by drawing on the psycho-sociological analysis of Douglas (1982) to outline the fit between health and defined cultural contexts. In so doing, he is articulating further the social theory positions that underpin the models of health promotion in the 1991 framework.

As with the 1991 framework, Beattie's (1993) work is based on two dimensions of conflict. The top-down paternalistic and bottom-up participatory mode of thought replaces the mode of intervention axis and is concerned with epistemology in terms of objective and subjective knowledge respectively. The focus of intervention axis is substituted for the focus of attention and, as with the former framework remains concerned with individual versus micro and macro population issues. The intersection of these axes enumerates four models of health in the same format as Figure 2.1.

The biopathological model of health has an individual focus of attention and operates from a positivistic, epistemological position where objective, rational and expert and paternalistic views on health dominate. Jones and Naidoo (2000) suggest that it underpins health persuasion techniques where the emphasis is on individuals taking responsibility for health-related behaviour, and this is consistent with the assertions of Naidoo and Wills (2000). Both models represent a 'conservative' (Beattie 1991: 184, 1993: 265; Jones and Naidoo 2000: 91) socio-political philosophy that translate in practice into minimal state intervention in all matters including health. The ecological model of health shares the same position on the mode of thought axis as the biopathological model but has a collective focus of attention. For Beattie (1991), legislative action for health, where the focus of intervention for the health of macro populations is determined by epidemiological data (Naidoo and Wills 2000), is informed by the ecological model of health. Both represent a reforming, traditional left wing (Beattie 1991, 1993) socio-political philosophy advocating legislative and policy interventions for public health improvement of the type described earlier when outlining the legislative action for health model of health promotion.

The biographical and communitarian models are philosophically humanistic and epistemologically interpretive. In equating health with individual and micro population empowerment and autonomy, Naidoo and Wills (2000) illustrate their conceptual fit with personal counselling for health and community development for health respectively. As the title suggests, the former links health with the active shaping of personal biographies. As with personal counselling for health, where the emphasis is on enhancing personal control of life and facilitating change on issues identified by the client (Naidoo and Wills 2000), the biographical model of health represents a liberal socio-political philosophy (Beattie 1991, 1993). In contrast, the latter is at the collective end of the focus of intervention axis. In common with community development for health, health is seen as a social experience achieved through emancipatory interventions and direct community action for change reflecting a radical but pluralistic socio-political philosophy (Beattie 1991, 1993).

When presented by Beattie (1993), the grid/group analysis framework of Douglas (1982) on divergent socio-cultural positions has the same fourfold structure as the Beattie (1991, 1993) frameworks. For Douglas, perception is shaped by cultural experiences and by bias associated with those experiences as a result of social interactions. The assumption is that the latter can be interpreted, sorted and reduced to defined social categories. Douglas (1982) achieves this via a two-dimensional grid/group analysis. The intersection of a high grid/low grid axis, symbolising levels of social order, hierarchy and personal control, with a high group/low group axis, symbolising both levels of social cohesion and inclusiveness, creates four social categories. Although these represent extreme views of social thought and behaviour Douglas contends that these can be used to classify the infinite range of social interactions.

The low grid/low group culture of individualism is demonstrated by people negotiating their life choices and actions and developing alliances and allows for individual mobility up and down the social scale. The high grid/low group culture of subordination represents a social position in which people are isolated and not part of a group; are relatively powerless and behave according to dictat. The high grid/high group culture of hierarchy/control is demonstrated when people act according to institutional processes and structures and social stratification, associated stability and security and respect for the social order. The low grid/high group culture of co-operation/factions is concerned with classifying social interactions in relation to group membership and forms of micro society in which only the external group boundary is clear.

POSTMODERNISM, METATHEORY AND BEATTIE'S FRAMEWORKS AS 'IDEAL TYPES'

Miller (1997) outlines the postmodern theoretical position in relation to nursing. No single theory or narrative can claim dominance or to have captured absolute truth because all are incomplete in a social theory world of multiplicities, indeterminacies, fragmentations and pluralities of small-scale situated knowledge influenced by cultures, traditions, values, ideologies and family life (Miller 1997). Postmodern theorists reject grand narrative and call for a multiplicity of paradigms, theories and methods to reflect the complexity of the discipline.

In line with this, Beattie's (1991, 1993) frameworks, via reference to the work of Douglas (1982), offer a multidimensional view of health promotion, health and cultural bias. In operating from a metatheoretical premise they embrace competing, dichotomous and incommensurable, but not mutually exclusive, models and philosophical perspectives. As described earlier, these models are ideologically, epistemologically and methodologically convergent and compatible at some points and divergent and contradictory at others. The frameworks then, in supplying contrasting metatheoretical assumptions, address Feyerabend's (1975) call for theoretical understanding through comparison, competition between alternatives and mutually incompatible positions and methodological pluralism. It is the process of this competition, where nothing is ever settled and where in this instance each model of health promotion, health and cultural bias within the frameworks act as an external standard of criticism for others, which contributes to the development of consciousness (Feyerabend 1975).

For the purpose of the book, Beattie's (1991, 1993) frameworks and the derived nursing health promotion framework for nursing in Chapter 5 represent sensitising analytical schemes (Turner 1987).

These are provisional theoretical constructions subject to change but which provide a structured basis for the development of a health promotion framework for nursing at the time of writing. They provide a starting point for generating testable theory and for preliminary conceptualisation about basic classes of variables. However, as factor-relating theories, which both classify and depict situations but which do not predict relationships or generate hypotheses, they cannot be theory tested in the traditional quantitative way. The frameworks are a form of analytical, as opposed to explanatory theory in expressing theoretical rather than empirical concerns (Fallding 1971).

Thus, the frameworks exist in abstract only and as such constitute 'ideal type' theories. Weber (1971) describes 'ideal types' as internally consistent theoretical devices that give unambiguous expression to conceptual relationships that accentuate aspects of reality. As 'ideal types', the health promotion frameworks are heuristic devices providing clearly stated general concepts that can facilitate the classification, comparison and appraisal of the research findings in relation to multiple perspectives and competing value and belief systems (Jary and Jary 1991). Although illuminating social phenomena, as untestable hypothetical constructions (Abercrombie *et al.* 1988) elements of the 'ideal type' are not always observable in reality. However, when applied herein as conceptual and diagnostic tools that guide analysis they enhance understanding and help establish the extent to which reality deviates from the ideal (Crotty 1996).

ARCHITECTURALLY COMPATIBLE FRAMEWORKS

A number of frameworks by other authors reflect essentially the same fourfold structural format of Beattie (1991, 1993). The variation in the use of the terms health education and health promotion simply reflect the different ways in which the authors use them and does not reflect the definitions of these concepts as advanced in Chapter 1. Preceding Beattie's (1991, 1993) work, while similarly aware of the plethora of approaches by other theorists and particularly interested in the relationship between the health educator and the client/client group, Nutbeam (1984) felt it important to construct a framework to support his categorisation of health education. Nutbeam intersects a locus of intervention variable with a locus of power variable to create four types of health education. The locus of intervention variable is a continuum of interventions that range from those at an individual level to those with a societal focus, while the locus of power variable identifies the power base from which the health educator is operating.

51

The health education types interrelate on one axis and are opposed on the other. Type A health education is individually centred but authoritarian and its intervention takes the form of prescribed behaviour change of a preventive nature by a health care professional on a one-to-one basis. Type B health education maintains the individual behavioural focus and one-to-one level of intervention, but in promoting the client's health, locus of control, independence and autonomy is non-authoritarian. Nutbeam cites the teacher–pupil relationship as a classic example of this type of health education. Type C and type D health education are community centred but again, like type A and type B, are divided by their modes of authority. The former aims to achieve community participation and change in line with a top-down professionally determined agenda through influencing either the community or the key protagonists within a community. Type D health education is conversely bottom-up with the initiative for action emanating from the community members and where the role of the health educator is to assist the community in identifying and meeting health needs. This is a variation on the Beattie (1991) theme but lacks reference to wider socio-political philosophy or theory and any real depth of analysis.

Like Beattie, Caplan (1993) also laments the lack of a more fundamental theoretical analysis by health promotion theorists in their models and frameworks. He also extols the importance of social theory for health education, but instead of adopting Beattie's (1991) structural map he advances Burrell and Morgan's (1979) theoretical map of social theory paradigms and organisational analysis as the definitive basis for a health education framework. He omits any reference to Beattie other than to an early 1984 paper.

Caplan's (1993) writing is a development of his unpublished MSc dissertation and his work with Holland (Caplan and Holland 1990), which in turn derives from Whittington and Holland's (1985) adaptation of Burrell and Morgan's theoretical map for social work. Caplan and Holland (1990) also took the view that models and theories of health education are predicated on inadequate theoretical foundations and advocated a broader understanding of social theory. Their theoretical map is largely the same as Caplan's (1993) in outlining four models of health education that relate to paradigms of social theory. The difference is in the use of some of the terminology. For example, Caplan and Holland's 'traditional health education' is referred to by Caplan as 'functionalist' and the term Marxist no longer accompanies radical structuralist health education.

Caplan (1993) is far more expansive than Caplan and Holland (1990). For example, the way in which they explain their health education models is more superficial, and their exposition of Marxist theory in relation to health education and what this would actually mean in practice is minimal. Caplan (1993) argues that the depth and rigour of Burrell and Morgan's (1979) theoretical map applied to health education enables not just epistemological and ideological scrutiny but also pragmatic assessment of the social focus and core concepts of the four models (or paradigms). He entitles these 'radical', 'radical structuralist', 'humanist' and 'functionalist' health education. As with Beattie (1991, 1993), they emerge from the intersection of the two fundamental social theory dimensions (although in this case it is the nature of social science and the nature of knowledge).

The operationalisation and application to health education of fundamental elements of theoretical discourse and elucidation of competing health education models again, like Beattie's work, juxtaposes models (paradigms) that are complementary at one level but contradictory at another. In effect Caplan is saying that the emergent models of health education are empirical manifestations of quintessential theoretical positions and structures. He argues that these need to be understood to grasp truly what models of health education represent. This level of understanding and explicit application of the framework to health education enables Caplan to articulate a proper analysis and a mapping of the core view of society, principal health determinants and the aims of each of the partially competing health education models. Unlike Burrell and Morgan, and unlike Beattie's view of the models in his framework, Caplan deems the models/paradigms not to be mutually exclusive at all levels.

Functionalist health education targets individual health-related attitudes and behaviours. It aims to change these in line with scientifically derived, objective facts and externally imposed medical goals to achieve self-regulation. This approach also modifies personal behaviour through enacting legislation and public policy engaging in social engineering, but within a framework of social conservatism and never so boldly as to threaten the political and socio-structural status quo. Caplan does not spell out exactly what he means by social engineering and he does not give explicit examples of legislative interventions within this paradigm but does emphasise the shaping of individual behaviour.

The use of legislative machinery and public policy, but for the purpose of radical change, is also a feature of radical structuralist health education. Here, the analysis of health determinants moves

53

away from individual behaviour and risk factors and on to the relationship between health and the inherent inequalities and exploitation of the capitalist economic and social class-based structure. Caplan applies this to health education circumspectly, suggesting that if operationalised it would address the conflicts and struggles of working people to improve material conditions and challenge capitalism. Unfortunately, he neither gives examples nor states methods of intervention other than to link health education to such initiatives. He does note that as an instrument of health education it can be employed by paradigms with epistemologically compatible but polarised views of the social world, and is thus not paradigm specific.

Caplan goes on to contend that perhaps the best way to achieve collective health gain is through radical social change but at a bottom-up micro-level. Radical health education is a means of harnessing community action through community development that aims to maximise community empowerment. This is facilitated by strengthening mutual aid and social support, self-help and participation engendering a sense of community control and autonomy on issues determined by the members of the community. He feels that in practice community development actually reflects a humanistic approach to health education and is an extension of social regulation as it operates within a framework of social consensus. The aims are stated as improving self-awareness and an understanding of others, of reflection and clarification of problems and of reshaping biographies in line with personal aspirations.

Writing at the same time as Caplan and Holland (indeed in the same journal) Taylor (1990) also undertook a theoretical mapping exercise. She also used Burrell and Morgan's (1979) work ostensibly as a means of elucidating the theoretical and philosophical assumptions of the radical structuralist, radical humanist, traditional functionalist and humanist models of health education. Taylor's (1990) short, descriptive article is devoted to outlining the models within the map that dovetail with those of Caplan and Holland (1990) and Caplan (1993), rather than critically examining the underpinning theory.

Hagquist and Starrin (1997) are interested in the application of models of health education to the school setting. Their framework of four models emanates from intersecting contextual and strategy for change dimensions. The traditional educational models are a top-down strategy for change within a narrow contextual framework. In schools this resembles traditional didactic classroom teaching, but on health education topics, where knowledge and facts are disseminated by school teachers to passive recipients. It is based on the assumption that individual children will make rational health-related behaviour choices in response to this input.

Modern educational models occupy the same narrow position on the contextual framework dimension as the traditional models and are also applied in the classroom setting, but their strategy for change is bottom-up. The difference here is the concentration on factors that influence behaviour, rather than on behaviour itself. Pupils become active participants and interventions are designed to encourage emotional development, social resistance, and to foster decision-making skills and build self-esteem.

Planner and empowerment models share a wide contextual framework but diverge on the strategy for change dimension. Planner models are top-down in that health education interventions aim to improve the overall school environment, links with the family and wider community. They are run for, rather than with or by, the pupils and are thus indirect in both pupil impact and involvement. Within the wider contextual framework empowerment models pursue a bottom-up strategy for change. Pupils are seen as partners in health education work, as capable of representing themselves, making decisions and influencing school policies and their collective relationship with adults and, for example, school committees are seen as a key issue. As an approach it resembles community activism and community development, which are concerned with collective self-determination, the use and control of local resources and mechanisms of power for micro-structural change.

Hagquist and Starrin's (1997) framework and its all-embracing orthogonal dimensions offers scope for analysis of health education models beyond their application to schools as it provides a framework by which alternative, competing approaches can be classified at different levels. Their work resembles, indeed could be a derivation of, Beattie's (1991) structural map of health promotion but it lacks the depth of his socio-political analysis and he is not cited by the authors.

CONCLUSION

Silva (1986) advances that of the numerous nursing studies that have used conceptual models as research frameworks, few have tested the underlying validity of their assumptions or propositions. Silva attributes this to a lack of investigator commitment and sees it as an impediment to the testing of nursing theory. The same criticism might also be levelled at the use of models and frameworks of health promotion. To offset this, Chapter 2 has identified and applied internal theory testing criteria to test the rigour and conceptual adequacy of Beattie's (1991), and by implication Piper and Brown's (1998a) and Piper's (2000, 2004, 2007a, 2007b) frameworks of health promotion models to help justify it as the general benchmark that underpins the specific nursing health promotion framework of this book. This chapter also advanced the complementary Beattie (1993) and Douglas (1982) structures to assist with the analysis, synthesis and philosophical contextualisation of this conceptual relationship. Having withstood the application of the internal theory testing criteria, the next step is to review the competing general health education and health promotion frameworks to test further Beattie's (1991) pre-eminent position; and this is the focus of Chapter 3.

LEARNING TRIGGERS

Having read Chapter 2, complete the learning triggers below to reinforce your understanding of the concepts that have been discussed:

- Define framework, theory and model and summarise the difference between them.
- Summarise the difference between factor-isolating; factor-relating; situation-relating; and situation-producing theory.
- Summarise the criteria that have been used to test the conceptual adequacy of health promotion frameworks.
- Summarise Beattie's (1991) health promotion framework and its inherent models.
- Identify the relationship between the frameworks and models of health, cultural bias and health promotion.
- Define postmodernism, metatheory and 'ideal types'.

GENERAL HEALTH EDUCATION AND HEALTH PROMOTION FRAMEWORK REVIEW

3

INTRODUCTION

This chapter presents and reviews the general (i.e. from outside of nursing) frameworks of health education and health promotion. In line with Guba and Lincoln's (1989) thinking, the purpose of the review is to sketch out and consider conceptual devices that might challenge Beattie's (1991) and thus Piper and Brown's (1998a) and Piper's (2000, 2004, 2007a, 2007b) work as the foundation of the health promotion framework for nursing advanced in Chapter 5. In effect this aspect of the literature review constitutes additional, and a form of triangulated, theory testing. The methodology used to guide the process, the rationale for the sequence of the health education/ promotion framework review and the context of the debate are also outlined.

LEARNING OUTCOMES

By reading this chapter, and completing the learning triggers at the end, the reader should have a better conceptual grasp of:

- the health promotion framework review methodology;
- health promotion frameworks that co-exist and compete with Beattie's (1991) (see Chapter 2) work in addition to those in Chapters 2 and 4;
- the limitations of the frameworks in relation to Beattie's (1991) work and the derived but specific nursing health promotion frameworks of Piper and Brown (1998a) and Piper (2000, 2004, 2007a, 2007b).

HEALTH EDUCATION/PROMOTION FRAMEWORK REVIEW METHODOLOGY

The review is based on an inclusive, structured and extensive search of electronic databases, grey literature (conference proceedings, discussion papers, organisation publications and unpublished work), hand searching of key books and journals and personally contacting contributors to the debate on health promotion frameworks. Although not exhaustive, the review selects key health promotion frameworks from the author's (Piper 2004) unpublished research to illustrate the tenor, character, nature and focus of the debate. The review includes health promotion frameworks however described that include two or more models of health education or health promotion, but other than this there were no additional exclusion criteria.

RATIONALE FOR THE SEQUENCE OF THE HEALTH EDUCATION/ PROMOTION FRAMEWORK REVIEW

The order in which the general health education and health promotion models and frameworks are presented and categorised is by formative theory building, discipline, more advanced theorising or by being high currency. In part this gives a sense of the history and chronology of how these devices and the debate evolved and developed. However, although the frameworks were constructed within an historical and a policy context, as can be seen there is no definitive link between framework sophistication and age of the work. As with Chapter 2, the variation in use of the terms health education and health promotion simply reflects the different ways in which the authors use them.

FORMATIVE HEALTH PROMOTION THEORY BUILDING

The early years of health promotion models and framework development are notable because of self-imposed narrow parameters, superficiality and descriptive work mostly lacking in a depth of analysis in general and in relation to wider social theory in particular.

Tuckett (1979) helped initiate the framework debate by advancing three analytically different but compatible strategies that he contends frames the range of health education activity. As can be seen below, the models within Tuckett's (1979) framework are all examples of top-down or professionally led interventions based on normatively determined health need. They do not reflect bottom-up individual or community empowerment models based on subjective perception of life experience and health needs. Health education was seen as:

- a branch of preventive medicine concerned to educate the public about health-related beliefs and risk-taking behaviour (for example, smoking, diet, exercise and safer sex);
- a way of getting the public to use health care facilities appropriately and effectively, the channelling of expectations to ensure compliance with what is available and the development of self-care strategies;
- education on topics such as sex, parenting skills and interpersonal relations to direct the public towards socially desirable and healthy behaviour.

Tuckett acknowledges that disease and disability might be influenced by socio-economic forces and that risk-taking behaviour may be due to low morale and poor self esteem as a result of limited life opportunities or dangerous and dirty jobs. Tuckett suggests that preventive health education might highlight these health determinants and influence public opinion towards pressing for political, economic and legislative change.

Draper *et al.* (1980) and Draper (1983)

Beattie (1991) congratulates Draper *et al.* (1980) and Draper (1983) for going beyond the traditional omnipresent medical model but he views their approaches to health education as essentially lists of information that health educators might transmit to the public. They are cited here as an example of a framework that fails to address to any great extent the relationship between models of health education and wider theoretical disputes (Beattie 1991).

Draper *et al.* (1980) outline three types of health education. In part these are a variation on Tuckett's (1979) and focus on:

- (Type 1) hygiene, human biology and the workings of the body and how to maintain its functioning;
- (Type 2) informing the public about the role, availability and appropriate use of health care resources and self-care strategies such as what action to take following an accident;
- (Type 3) health policy. Here Draper *et al.* go further than Tuckett (1979) and contend that to restrict health education to the first two types is irresponsible, and the majority of their article is given over to type 3.

Type 3 health education is seen as an extension of the public health tradition. It seeks to highlight how health choices are shaped by the wider physical and socio-economic environment and by European, national, regional and local policies. Draper *et al.* lambaste the preoccupation with indiscriminate economic growth, vested financial interests and the creation of an over pressurised society. They highlight that the way that goods are produced, as well as what is produced, are important health issues and contend that the creation of wealth may be at the expense of health. It is interesting to note that, although not explicitly referred to, Draper *et al.*'s (1980) work was published just after Margaret Thatcher had formed a radical and fervently monetarist UK Conservative government in 1979.

Type 3 health education both informs and encourages the public to adopt environmentally and ecologically sustainable patterns of social behaviour, while endeavouring to influence legislative and institutional policies so as to make healthy choices easier. In addition to the models outlined the article also refers to community development as an approach to health education but no rationale is offered for its exclusion from their framework.

Much of Draper's (1983) expanded five types of health education equate with his earlier collaborative work and again balances the responsibility individuals have for leading a healthy lifestyle against the social and environmental determinants of health. In the latter paper the political and environmental issues are sub-divided into separate models with the environment including sustainable economic growth, green issues and alternative ways of living and means of fulfilment. Education about power and accountability in society, inequality, the special needs of sections of the community (for example, those with a disability, ethnic groups, single parents) and about the need for health protective policies and legislation comes under the heading of politics of health. The fifth and final variety of health education in Draper's (1983) framework is prosaically entitled 'about health education itself'. In seeking to educate about the outcomes, effectiveness and organisation of health education in relation to human ecology it is essentially a process of evaluation and dissemination.

Dorn (1981)

Dorn's three types of health education are of interest specifically because they are summarised in relation to theories of knowledge, i.e. wider theoretical disputes. The effects model has a conservative morality approach to value-free and common sense health knowledge. It aims to influence people individually and collectively through the use of didactic and affective methods. The structuralist model has a radical morality approach to knowledge. It works across the spectrum of personality, culture, language and the economy, struggling to overthrow dominant political philosophies and beliefs. The active model is a material approach to knowledge that, as a synthesis of the first two types of health education, focuses on the development between health education theory and practice and their impact on the material determinants of social health. Dorn endeavours to translate these into health education for young people but with minimal success due to the brevity of the framework, the ideological distinction between the types and what this means for practice.

Burkitt (1983)

Reference to Burkitt's (1983) work helps to illustrate the complexity, expansive nature and yet superficiality of some of the frameworks. Burkitt integrates seven approaches to health education with seven models of health and concomitant sites of action, agents/disciplines and therapies. The models are not seen as mutually exclusive, as a combination of two or more may be used and they may additionally operate at primary, secondary and tertiary points of intervention. The pathological/medical model is as for preventive/medical models, as described later and in more detail by other authors in this chapter.

The emphasis of the socio-psychological and psycho-sociological models of health are individual and group interpersonal interactions and cultural norms and influences, but their therapies and approaches to health education differ. The former is target group-based and uses social planning and community development techniques for social and welfare support. The psycho-sociological model uses individual or small group counselling and group therapy techniques to build self-awareness, self-esteem, social skills and sensitivity.

Ecological health is associated with people in their environment and with the community as its site of action. As with the preceding models the key agents and disciplines are education and health and social care professionals. It includes the use of pressure groups and the therapy is listed as legislation and single-issue activity on environmental problems. The health education approaches utilised are mass media campaigns and awareness-raising to change public opinion and law enforcement.

The traditional model of health uses healers (faith, diet, herbal) as its agents and their disciplines and therapy to correct imbalances in the body. It is information-based and about highlighting what the therapies can offer. The traditional Chinese medicine Taoist model of health is similar across all categories but broadens the site of action to the relationship of humans to their world and the balance of chi, yin and yang. It is more spiritual/vocational with a master–student relationship and a life path to follow.

Finally, the socialist model of health acts from a social class and collective action perspective and targets workers of the world. The agents and disciplines of change are the politically conscious leaders, Socialist/Marxist economics, and Burkitt cites Maoist China. The therapy is social change and economic equality via political education, highlighting inequality, facilitating trade union activity and other class-based confrontation. Burkitt introduces a magnitude of philosophies, social theories and social movements but their substance is glossed over, many questions are left unanswered and there is no real depth to any of the models of health. For example, Burkitt does not explain the agent and discipline of Maoist China in relation to health education.

Anderson (1984)

Anderson's work is cited because it provides an overview of health promotion for the World Health Organization. Anderson (1984) maintained that there is no neat classification system and that it is ambitious to think one could be devised given the diversity of activities that fall under this heading. He nevertheless goes on to identify and give examples of three categories of health promotion. These are entitled:

- individual or group practices;
- measures designed to support health promotion by individuals and groups;
- changes in the environment designed to result in a direct improvement in health.

The first category refers to activities that might be undertaken by individuals or groups to enhance their own health and that of others, rather than those undertaken in response to disease. These include the gamut of health-related behaviours, hobbies, personal development and involvement in community groups and community action for local social and environmental change. Examples of outcomes of intervention include improved health, welfare and social provision or reducing noise, traffic and air pollution.

The second health promotion category contains sub-categories A and B. The education and training measures of sub-category A are designed to develop health-related decision-making, social and coping skills. Sub-category B is where individuals or groups endeavour to improve both their physical and social environment. It takes the form of community campaigning and action on issues such as play areas for children, cycling and jogging paths, provision of leisure facilities and meeting places for the community, and improving access to health, welfare and social services. Health gain for category three stems from enacting health protective legislation to reduce the health-damaging effects of the environment and health enhancing environmental measures. The issues might include noise pollution, poor-quality housing, poor working conditions and road safety, and improvements to the physical and architectural environment.

Later in the same work Anderson goes on to describe four categories of activity that may maintain or improve health. These equate with the three categories previously identified. The difference is that sub-categories A and B of the earlier category two become two distinct categories entitled 'educational and training activities' and 'changes in the environment designed to facilitate the promotion of health by individuals or groups'. Category three becomes category four with a different title (changes in the environment to be of direct benefit to the public) but with the same substance as described before.

Tones (1986) cites Anderson when noting the conceptual confusion surrounding health promotion. This can be seen by the lack of clarity and overlap between the aims and methods of Anderson's categories of health promotion and is exacerbated by the lack of consistency when redefining the categories later in his work. Most interestingly, none of the categories outlined refer in any significant way to the dominant medical model, mass media and information-giving approaches to health promotion.

Keeley-Robinson (1984)

Health education within adult education forms the context for Keeley-Robinson's review of models of health education, and warrants mention as the work is also applied to health visitor (public health nursing) training and practice in Chapman and Slavin (1985). Both incorporate either the preventive (Keeley-Robinson 1984) or the equivalent medical (Chapman and Slavin 1985) and the educational, community development and self-empowerment models (Chapman and Slavin use the descriptor self-development interchangeably with self-empowerment) and fit with others of the same nomenclature. For the political economy (Keeley-Robinson) and radical social action

(Chapman and Slavin) models read radical (Tones 1981, 1986) and radical-political (Tones *et al.* 1990), as the differences are merely semantic.

Seymour (1984)

Seymour classifies health education by:

- traditional;
- educational;
- new wave

interventions and provides an extremely concise explanation of each category. The first two are briefly defined in language and meaning compatible with those of others described elsewhere herein and new wave health education strands community action and legislative/environmental activities. Seymour's work is of interest because it adopts something of an anti-theoretical pragmatic position. He contends that the theoretical debate has done nothing to clarify the practice of health education/promotion and has merely compounded any conceptual confusion. In alluding to the classic theorist/practitioner tension he maintains that the theoretical constructions of academics do not reflect the reality of practice. In offering a pragmatic solution, Seymour's stance is somewhat contradictory as his article engages in theorising and, as Rawson and Grigg (1988) point out, he adds to the increasingly overwhelming number of models of health education.

Massey and Carnell (1987)

Massey and Carnell put forward a framework of health education for schools that at first glance might be of interest to school nurses, hence its inclusion. However, closer scrutiny reveals a cursory description of the models entitled:

- medical (preventive)
- educational
- pastoral (self-empowerment)
- radical.

The distinction between the models, for example, the educational and pastoral, lacks clarity and there is no exploration of organisational or structural interventions. They are criticised by French and Adams (1988) for their lack of reference to published work on health education theory and for the shallowness of their review of models.

Abelin (1987)

Abelin takes a different tack in basing his framework of six interacting approaches to health promotion and disease prevention on factors that determine health. He maintains that there is no one best approach and that the challenge is to identify the best combinations. The identification of high-risk individuals in terms of disease prevention, risk factor management, behaviour change and encouraging the use of services (for example, immunisation and screening), which may involve outreach and referral in the developing world, is the domain of the medical and related services approach.

Health education consists of the transmission of knowledge and the development of concomitant values, attitudes and life-skills to enable life-choices and resistance to unwanted social pressures. This may be of relevance to school nurses as schools are particularly emphasised as the key setting for these interventions. Community-oriented health promotion is pretty much as for Beattie's (1991) community development and community social work techniques, although these are not defined precisely by Abelin.

The environmental health approach is essentially public health measures to do with health protection from pollution and health hazards, environmental regulation and surveillance, food processing and food importation. Abelin distinguishes this approach from health-orientated legislation that embraces wider legal and regulatory frameworks to enable the promotion of health. This is via regulating professional bodies and advertising, legislation on employment, housing and transport and government fiscal and monetary policy. The final approach, occupational health, is as for environmental health but specifically applied to the workplace.

Epp (1987)

As with Lalonde (1974) and the 'health field concept', the contribution of a national politician always merits consideration, particularly as in this case it was at the famous International Conference on Health Promotion in Ottawa, Canada in 1986. In its published form Epp (1987), the Minister of National Health and Welfare for Canada, outlines a framework for health promotion. Against a backdrop of demographic and social change the three major health challenges of reducing inequalities in health, increasing prevention and developing individual coping strategies were synthesised with health promotion mechanisms and strategies for implementation to create a framework for health promotion. Epp (1987) maintains that the potential for health promotion outcomes of this multi-strand, inter-related framework surpasses what could be achieved by single strategies and mechanisms. The mechanisms of:

- self-care;
- mutual aid;
- healthy environment

constitute health promotion models within the larger framework.

The self-care mechanism refers to the preventive health-related beliefs, attitudes and behaviour of individuals and when opera-tionalised means encouraging healthy choices. Collective effort and support and sharing ideas and experiences at a family, neighbourhood and self-help group level on health concerns is the domain of the mutual aid model, with informal networks explicitly recognised as fundamental to health promotion. The third mechanism for promoting health is the creation of healthy environments by modifying socio-economic and physical structures and through the use of health and social legislation on health, education, transport, the workplace and ecological issues.

Within the framework there are three strategies for implementing the health promotion mechanisms. Fostering public participation aims to help individuals cope with and assert control over health deter-minants through self-help, counselling, education and information and helping people make use of services. Strengthening community health services aims to expand community-based provision and orientate them more toward disease prevention and health promotion focusing on particular challenges to health. In practice, this might mean targeting services to meet the needs of those materially disadvantaged, involving communities in service planning, alliances between health and social services and fostering self-care, mutual aid and the creation of healthy environments.

The third strategy for promoting health is co-ordinating healthy public policy to facilitate the implementation of the health promotion mechanisms. The aim is equality in health experience and making healthy choices easier choices. It is acknowledged that there is the potential for conflict between, for example, the vested interests of some in manufacturing industry and those for whom the focus is solely public-policy change for environmental gain. Clearly Epp's (1987) framework was designed as a pragmatic tool and is concerned with health-promotion policy development and application, rather than detailed scrutiny of competing theoretical positions and reflexive analysis.

Minkler (1989)

Minkler proffers Epp's (1987) framework for health promotion, cited above, as one of two *directions* for health education, each of which reflects a unique vision of health promotion (no precise definition is offered of health education or health promotion or of their differences). The first direction is mostly a means to achieve individual behaviour change and risk modification. While acknowledging that lifestyle and health-related behaviour are important influences on health, Minkler links this direction to the capitalist model of consumer choice. He strongly critiques the way in which it blames individuals for their self-imposed risk and ignores material inequality and the socio-economic framework that shapes choice and which is a major health determinant. These oversights are what attract Minkler to the alternative direction of the framework for health promotion as it puts forward reducing inequality as the primary challenge, a situation that persists in the UK (Department of Health 2002b).

Pederson et al. (1991)

Pederson *et al.*'s conceptual framework describes the role of legislation and education in reducing exposure to passive smoking. Their framework incorporates individual and socio-political variables that influence compliance with restrictions. The authors cite the use of motor vehicle seatbelts as an example of where legislation and education have previously been used as the two strategies to influence health-related behaviour. This is a highly focused, topic-specific and intentionally narrow, top-down exploration of what health educators and policy makers can do to obtain the compliance of smokers with the enactment and implementation of legislation controlling smoking. As the seatbelt example illustrates, as a way of working it has potential for transfer to other areas of health promotion.

TOPIC-SPECIFIC HEALTH EDUCATION/PROMOTION FRAMEWORKS

Hornsey (1982)

The distinguishing feature of Hornsey's (1982) fourfold framework of:

- medical;
- educational;

- developmental;
- socio-political

models of health education is its application to a particular phase of life, i.e. pre-retirement, and thus client group. The ubiquitous medical model, which Hornsey describes as 'victim-blaming' and authoritarian, equates with the preventive model and this, together with the adult educational model essentially occupy the same territory of those described by others herein. The participatory methods of the educational model involve discussion, sharing experiences, group interaction and support, and means of discovering ways to incorporate healthy behaviours into daily life with the philosophy of enjoying life to the full. The developmental model is similarly concerned to develop the skills of older adults so they can determine their own physical, mental and emotional health needs and goals and take appropriate action to fulfil them. However, it also concentrates on personal relationships, life changes and the sharing of both problems and personal resources within the context of pre-retirement groups.

The socio-political model moves the focus from individual action to the socio-economic and political determinants of health. It aims to mobilise the community to act as a pressure group from the perspective of community need to achieve social change, material gain and increased health or welfare service provision. This descriptive framework helpfully illustrates how these models can be applied to a specific client group, but there is a lack of a considered critique of what each more fundamentally represents; any detailed development of the models; or rationale for why they are more appropriate for retirement than competing published work.

Jones (1990)

The work of Jones, using the framework of Des Jarlais and Friedman (1987), reflects a time in the UK when there was a strong focus on HIV prevention. The strategies of Jones (1990) for preventing HIV transmission among intravenous drug users are not just topic-specific but also focus on a particular client group. There are six preventive mechanisms of intervention, concerned with:

- Maintenance and detoxification programmes that include encouraging the cessation of sharing drug paraphernalia, moving onto oral drug use and towards abstinence, flexible prescribing and supervised withdrawal from illicit drug use.

- The provision of sterile needles and syringes and other harm-minimisation equipment and practices.
- Education in a variety of settings (schools, prisons, etc.) using a range of methods. These range from didactic traditional mass media campaigns and behavioural and cultural interventions to self-empowerment and community action, but here Jones lacks clarity and detail in his exposition of the different approaches. Counselling and HIV antibody testing also come under the heading of education.
- Changing relationships. This includes mechanisms four, five and six. The former emphasises the need to change relationships between drug users and suggests that this might be achieved by self-help groups, organising drug users' or partners' organisations, and changing social norms to ones where risk-reduction behaviour is supported. The latter two emphasise changing social relationships between drug users and society and those that encourage intravenous use.

Overall Jones focuses on concrete examples of practice in relation to HIV, intravenous drug use and the analytical framework and remains within the narrow confines of prevention. He does not concern himself with detailed theoretical exposition or theoretical precision.

McEwan and Bhopal (1991)

McEwan and Bhopal are also interested in the application of a framework to health promotion on AIDS with young people. Although there is no broader conceptual exploration of the framework they critique four models of health promotion that fit with those of Beattie (1991). These are:

- policy development
- information-giving
- self-empowerment
- collective action.

The policy development approach achieves environmental change through legislation, policy, fiscal and economic intervention and can help create a climate that assists with access to services, legislates against prejudice and stigma and creates national curriculum initiatives.

Information-giving is noted as the dominant form of HIV/AIDS health promotion. Individual sexual behaviour is regarded as a matter of personal choice and preference and the assumption is that raising awareness and knowledge levels on HIV/AIDS via factual and imaginative campaigns using the media, leaflets and formal educational intervention will trigger the adoption of safer sexual practices in young people. McEwan and Bhopal (1991) note that although increased knowledge levels are achieved, the success of this approach in changing behaviour is poor.

Self-empowerment is concerned to facilitate personal choice and decision-making, self-determination and control over life and sexual health. It involves personal reflection and clarification of values and beliefs, the development of life-skills, confidence and self-esteem and the ability to resist peer pressure. An example of intervention cited is peer group teaching on HIV. The collective action approach is similarly concerned with empowerment but at the community level. Like policy development social, political, economic and cultural influences are seen as the key determinants of health but here the community drives the health promotion agenda. The use of the term community is not restricted to a residential geographical community but may mean, for example, a school or the gay community. Bottom-up collective action initiatives may consist of lobbying against stigma, prejudice and inequality or may include the development of self-help groups.

Franzkowiak and Wenzel (1994)

Franzkowiak and Wenzel's conceptual framework is similarly concerned with AIDS health promotion for young people. They describe the three principle strategies for health promotion:

- advocacy of policies;
- developing strong alliances and social support systems;
- empowering people.

These are noteworthy in that they are derived from the World Health Organization's work specifically on promoting health in developing countries. Although offering greater breadth and depth and using different nomenclature, Franzkowiak and Wenzel essentially cover the same terrain as McEwan and Bhopal (1991).

Nevertheless, it is worth flagging up that advocacy of policies has a number of elements. First, it is concerned to educate people irrespective of age, gender, social class or religious belief. Second, as individual health-related behaviour is viewed as a reflection of socio-economic forces, the lobbying of local, regional and national politicians and political organisations to achieve political action to address this is suggested. Pressure to ensure adequate resource (budgetary) allocation and the enacting of existing legal rights (for example under the United Nations Declaration of Human Rights) are also advanced as methods to meet the needs of people.

Developing strong alliances and support systems is about strengthening public-sector collaboration and alliances and an erosion of each sector pursuing solely its own objectives in favour of developing social networks, support and organisations within communities. Empowering people represents a synthesis of McEwan and Bhopal's (1991) self-empowerment and collective action approaches. Franzkowiak and Wenzel (1994) categorise this as a lifestyle approach and it forms the emphasis governing their thoughts on health promotion strategies. They highlight sexuality and concepts of body, reproduction, gender roles and risk behaviour as target areas for intervention and identify goals and primary and secondary target audiences.

PSYCHOLOGY AND SOCIAL MARKETING

Winett (1995) outlines a framework for programmes of health promotion and disease prevention. His contention is that the marginal effectiveness of some programmes is due to their failure to address the influence of environmental factors on health-related behaviour. Hence, Winett highlights the need to integrate theories and models for behaviour change with programme development at individual, group, organisation, community and institutional levels of intervention. Winett's (1995) six-category framework operates at a technical and applied level using the social marketing language of product, price, place and promotion (product promotion). His work is referred to as the social marketing approach, which is an acknowledged way of health promotion working and nurses need an awareness of it.

Health indicators determined by epidemiological data on causality and risk is the first category of Winett's (1995) framework, which also takes account of national priorities and goals for health (category two). These in turn are shaped by mortality, morbidity and health-related behaviour data. The fifth and sixth categories are the marketing plan, which is given particular emphasis, and the mechanics of implementation but it is categories three (methods) and four (approach) that are of particular interest herein. The methods of the framework are listed as health promotion, health protection and preventive services, which are integrated with primary, secondary and tertiary prevention. Despite the sophistication of the work, the emphasis is on essentially top-down interventions. These range from individuals taking responsibility for behaviour modification to health policy and programme development and legislation creating an environment conducive to catalysing professionally predetermined change.

ADVANCED AND HIGH-CURRENCY HEALTH EDUCATION/PROMOTION THEORY BUILDING

Although in 1981 Tones considered it difficult to define health education concisely and with precision, the identification of four overlapping and coexisting but philosophically different approaches to health education was the start of his significant, theoretically advanced and enduring contribution to the debate. The complexity of his framework has developed (Tones 1986; Tones *et al.* 1990; and Tones and Tilford 1994, 2001) but Beattie (1991) noted the importance of Tones' 1981 paper.

The education approach (Tones 1981, 1986) combines the provision of information of health risks with the sharing, exploring and clarifying of beliefs and values and an understanding of the implications of behaviour change in response to the health information. The aim is to achieve informed and free choice, and the methods, with young people for example, may include social skills training and development on issues such as 'safer sex' to facilitate decision-making and assertiveness. Tones appreciates that a person's life experience, role models, social and thus socio-economic context may impede informed and genuinely free choice, as may addiction to drugs, and that the provision of good advice may well be ignored.

The preventive (Tones 1981) or traditional (Tones 1986) approaches are based on the assumption that individual health-related behaviour such as diet, smoking or a lack of exercise are a precursor to disease. As the name suggests, the aim is to prevent disease and disability by encouraging, and at times coercing, people to lead a 'healthy' lifestyle and stop or modify elements of their lifestyle that are deemed unhealthy. Tones (1981) divides preventive health education into primary, secondary and tertiary categories as per Box 1.5 in Chapter 1.

Radical health education (Tones 1981, 1986) moves the focus on health determinants away from individual health-related behaviour to socio-economic and structural factors. Poor health experience is attributed to material inequality and disadvantage and, as with Draper *et al.* (1980), the health-damaging effects of a preoccupation with the relentless pursuit of increased productivity and economic growth. Instead of regaling individuals to eat the right foods, intervention needs to influence government policy to ensure that healthy food is readily accessible and affordable to all and raise public consciousness about social disadvantage and inequality and the need for government action to address this.

Approach to self-empowerment (Tones 1981), referred to as an alternative approach to the previous three, employs four strategies to empower individuals and facilitate choice. The first strategy aims to influence beliefs and attitudes towards deferred gratification and the changing of health-damaging behaviour. The second and third strategies aim to improve both individual perceptions of autonomy and control in life and health (internal locus of control) and self-esteem. The fourth strategy is not made explicit but may be the reference to social skills training in such areas as assertiveness, effective communication and feeling positive as part of enhancing a persons self-esteem. These models remain in Tones (1986) but self-empowerment is advanced as the central facilitating aspect of health promotion. In addition, and importantly, given the framework of the book in Chapter 5, Tones contends that the philosophically dissimilar and conflicting models are nevertheless not necessarily mutually exclusive.

Like Tones (1986), Tones *et al.* (1990) advance the preventive, radical-political and self-empowerment approaches to health education. Tones and Tilford (1994) pursue the same pattern but slightly modify the descriptors to preventive, radical and empowerment and give them greater depth and sophistication. They expand empowerment beyond self-empowerment to a concept embodying preventive, radical and educational models as subordinate elements. This remains the case in Tones and Tilford (2001) who propose the educational, preventive and empowerment models. The latter is again seen as a means to remedy the deficiencies of the first two and as an approach that now subsumes radical intervention by going beyond individual self-empowerment to include the empowerment of communities. It is considered radical in the sense that it challenges the narrow preventive model (Tones and Tilford 2001).

These frameworks reflect an interesting development of emphasis, yet the key themes remain constant. Self-empowerment strongly comes through as a primary aim of health education, but for Adams and Pintus (1994), in the earlier work, issues of freedom of choice and rationality are not addressed and its social function is not made explicit. Of equal pertinence is the absence of the concept of community empowerment, of working with and facilitating social health gain determined by the community from a bottom-up perspective. These are a feature of the later work with radical intervention discussed in relation to public health, raising peoples consciousness in relation to their plight and community empowerment (Tones and Tilford 2001).

French and Adams (1986, 1988) and French (1990)

The apparent confusion surrounding the nature of health education led French and Adams (1986) to propose their Tri-phasic map representing the start of their valuable input into the debate. The map is based on an analysis and synthesis of published theoretical models of health education and takes account of the relationship between its elements. It is intentionally hierarchical with a developmental methodological continuum of progressive degrees of empowerment and autonomy. The aims, ideological beliefs and values, the component parts and emphasis of the

- collective action;
- self-empowerment;
- behavioural change

models of health education are as for those of French and Adams (1988), with which the map shares strengths and limitations.

Unlike previously cited authors, French and Adams (1988) state that socio-economic influences are the major determinants of health, and individual health-related behaviour the least significant. As a result, they place the collective action model at the top of a three-model hierarchy followed in order of importance by self-empowerment and behavioural change. The collective action model defines health as a social product and aims for health gain through community-driven action on environmental, social and economic factors. Self-empowerment health education takes a bio-psycho-social holistic view of health and is for self-discovery and personal growth through reflection, clarification and life-skills development.

The behavioural change model, for optimum individual physical functioning is based on the assumption that health-related decisions are made rationally, and that information on health risks will achieve behavioural modification and compliance through favourably influencing the decision-making process. This brief article helpfully sketches out the aims of each model and the beliefs and values they hold on health, humanity, society and education. Examples of methods and evaluation criteria are provided but it is really no more than a summary and overview of their salient features.

French (1990) critiques and reconstructs his earlier descriptive work with Adams (French and Adams 1986). His stated primary purpose is to define the role of health education within health promotion. However, unlike Naidoo and Wills (2000) and the wider view as discussed in Chapter 1, what is most interesting is his contention that behaviour change, disease prevention and disease management should be divorced from health education and viewed as part of health promotion. The underlying principles and nature of health education are concisely spelled out and represent the content of the category identified within health promotion, and clear emphasis is given to empowerment as a central feature of health education, but there is minimal discussion and detail of the other categories.

French helpfully differentiates between community participation and community empowerment. The former can simply mean pursuing predetermined behaviour change in a community setting but can also reflect more empowering processes when community led. It is presented as an approach spanning the interdependent elements of French's non-hierarchical framework of health promotion. This encompasses disease management and disease prevention, which is seen as distinct from health education and the politics of health.

Community empowerment is an enabling approach that fosters increased control, or at least a perception of increased control over community events. A sub-category of community empowerment is social action that is combative action by the community to generate their own power base and to achieve their aims. French aligns this with radical-political ideology and to health promotion and thus outside the remit of health education. French's (1990) framework is considered for use in perioperative nursing by Snape (2000) but she concludes by questioning its practicality and appropriateness.

HIGH CURRENCY HEALTH EDUCATION/PROMOTION FRAMEWORKS

The following frameworks of Ewles and Simnett (2003) and Naidoo and Wills (2000) are high currency in that they are probably the most well known in nursing. To all intents and purposes their five approaches to health education/promotion, albeit with some minor difference of emphasis and terminology, are interchangeable. There is consensus among the authors that health promotion intervention is multi-faceted and utilises the various approaches depending on circumstances and need. They also contend that the approaches not only co-exist but in practice overlap and are complementary.

Ewles and Simnett (2003) summarise five approaches to intervention. Both the medical and behaviour change approaches aim to prevent disease and disability. The former aims to achieve this through promoting the uptake of preventive medical interventions such as immunisation. The latter through trying to get people to adopt a healthy lifestyle and comply with all the traditional messages in relation to smoking, eating, drinking and exercise. The educational approach follows that of Tones (1981), and bottom-up client-centred health promotion is about individual and collective empowerment and facilitating the client's health agenda. This may vary from setting up self-help groups to wider concerns of a community, although examples are not given of what constitutes community initiatives. Societal change aims to restructure the environment to enable healthier choices to be easier choices through political or social action to influence policy makers. This is both at a macro government policy level on health determinants and health inequalities, and at a micro institutional level, for example health promoting policies of schools and hospitals.

The five approaches of Naidoo and Wills (2000) follow the same pattern, nomenclature (for the most part) and have the same aims, methods and outcomes as Ewles and Simnett (2003). The difference is in the expanded and more detailed description of the aims and methods of each approach by Naidoo and Wills who, unlike Ewles and Simnett, also suggest brief evaluatory criteria, and in the substitution of the term empowerment for client centred.

Tannahill (1990) and Downie *et al.* (1990 and 1996)

Tannahill's (1985) and Downie *et al.*'s (1990, 1996) framework is similarly well known. In attempting to resolve any semantic confusion and oversimplification surrounding health promotion their work takes account of overlap between the methods of intervention, preventive and positive objectives, and is offered as an inclusive framework for strategic development and implementation. Much of the original article (Tannahill 1985) is devoted to meanings and definitions. This is also a feature of the later writing as the authors are critical of the glib use of the term health promotion and the lack of conceptual clarity offered by others and yet the model is pragmatically outlined with relative brevity. This leads Adams and Pintus (1994) to criticise it as a sound-bite model.

The point of departure for Tannahill (1985) is the three overlapping macro categories of:

- health education
- prevention
- health protection.

Here health education is a process of communication to improve individual and collective health and prevent illness through influencing knowledge, attitudes and behaviour of members of the community and power holders. This is linked to empowerment (although this relationship is not fully expanded upon) and is promulgated as a participative two-way process (bottom-up as well as top-down). Prevention is divided into four elements but is in effect primary, secondary and tertiary health education, and health protection is both traditional public health interventions and wider regulatory and legislative controls to prevent disease and promote health.

From these three domains stem a further four areas for intervention generated by overlapping spheres; health promotion thus consists of seven domains. The first three are as described above, but when listed as part of the seven, Tannahill stresses that domain one does not overlap with other spheres despite the diagram suggesting otherwise. The fourth domain is the point of overlap between one and two and is preventive education for the public and professionals alike. Domain five is preventive health protection, which includes legislation to enforce compliance, and six is health protection health education with a positive focus, which Tannahill relates to lobbying for local needs. The synthesis of the three dominant spheres of activity is the seventh domain that is preventive health protection health education, and this draws on a combination of the methods cited.

Downie *et al.* (1996) have slightly refashioned the 1985 framework but they are essentially interchangeable and the domains relate to each other. This re-fashioning is accompanied by equally elaborate language in 1990. For example, the fourth domain is health education for preventive health protection and the seventh is health education aimed at positive health protection, but this is simplified in 1996.

Rather than offering clarification, Tannahill (1985) is engaging in a play on words (Rawson 2002); applying simplistic semantic boundaries onto a complex philosophical debate in a naively pragmatic way, and his conflation of the issue is creating further conceptual confusion (Rawson and Grigg 1988). While essentially concerned to outline what happens in practice, this descriptive model does not provide a rationale for why or when to select one approach in preference to another (Naido and Wills 2000). These arguments are equally pertinent to Downie et al. (1990) and Downie et al. (1996). In addition, there is no real attempt to make explicit the relationship between the models within the framework.

It is interesting to note Naidoo and Wills' (2000) assertion that this model is widely accepted by health care professionals, and Jowett (1992) and McBean (1992) have no hesitation in recommending it for use by community nurses despite the limitations outlined herein. This is interesting for the following reasons. First, Tannahill's (1985) model, and its subsequent development with others, seems to have received unparalleled criticism. Second, for example although Adams and Pintus (1994) are right to conclude that the model does not address the structural and root determinants of health, their assertion that this reflects Tannahill's medical background may be the magnet for this level of scrutiny. Third, what is missing from the debate is an acknowledgement that medical model interventions may be entirely appropriate for medical professionals or at least that this issue is worthy of further exploration (Rawson 2002).

In addition, and in the context of planning, Tannahill (1990) outlines three health education categories:

- disease-orientated
- risk factor-orientated
- health-orientated.

The theoretical foundations of these models are sufficiently explored to justify their inclusion here and they are presented in his collaborative writing (Downie et al. 1990, 1996) as a framework of health education orientations that reinforce theory in a practical way.

The first category aims to prevent mortality and morbidity from specific diseases, such as coronary heart disease or a type of cancer, and success is measured by achieving predetermined targets. These form the focus for an expert-led preventive health education programme to reduce risk factors in individuals by getting them to change or modify their behaviour. The risk factor-orientated category is similar in so far as it uses the same methods of intervention and success criteria, but different in that rather than being disease-specific it aims to reduce risk factors such as smoking that contribute to multiple disease aetiology.

Health-orientated health education transcends diseases and risk factors and is holistically orientated towards key groups (for example, school children) and key settings (for example schools). It is multi-disciplinary in its approach and uses various methods that can be tailored to the group or setting. It takes account of socio-economic variables, social pressures and the health needs defined by the client group. The outcomes go beyond just trying to prevent unhealthy behaviour and are about the development of life-enhancing skills, self-esteem, autonomy and thus empowerment. It aims then, to promote positive health and prevent illness. Downie *et al.* (1990, 1996) drop the key groups/key settings orientations and link the category to community development (somewhat tenuously) but otherwise dovetail with Tannahill (1990). The intentionally narrow scope of the framework means that models of health promotion that attempt to modify structures and environmental determinants of health are omitted.

Ecology (1988–96)

Unlike other descriptors that are merely means of semantic and technical classification, ecology has more overt ideological connotations and has subsequently been left until last as this makes it stand apart from the other groupings. McLeroy *et al.* (1988, 1992) propose an extremely comprehensive ecological framework of health promotion that targets individual and socio-environmental factors. This was constructed in response to the 'victim-blaming' lifestyle approach of traditional health promotion solely emphasising individual responsibility for health-damaging behaviour and ignoring socio-economic influences.

The framework of McLeroy *et al.* (1988) identifies the five strategies for health promotion:

- intrapersonal factors
- interpersonal processes
- institutional factors
- community factors
- public policy.

McLeroy *et al.* (1992) integrate these with change processes, under-pinning theories and models, targets of change and strategies and skills. The intrapersonal ecological level relies on psychological theories of change. It utilises education, mass- and social-marketing approaches and skills development to increase knowledge and change health-related attitudes, values and behaviours and improve self-esteem. Psychosocial theory underpins the interpersonal level that aims to change social norms and enhance social networks and support, as these directly influence values, beliefs, health and social behaviour, sense of personal identity and are the key social resource.

Intervention at the institutional (McLeroy *et al.* 1988) or organisational (McLeroy *et al.* 1992) level concentrates on organisational culture, structure and processes, leadership and management styles and incentive programmes to support behaviour change. The community level is about community empowerment through use of community development, community coalition and conflict strategies. It targets local power structures, the local economic and resource base, neighbourhood organisations and community competencies. The change processes of the public policy level are political. Health gain is achieved through changes in legislation and regulation and public policy development, advocacy and analysis.

Stokols' (1996) intention is to translate social ecology as an overarching framework, where ecology can be defined as the study of the interrelationship between organisms and environment, into guidelines for health promotion in the community. Stokols notes the shift in prominence from individual health-related behavioural interventions to those of a community and environmental nature reflecting the increased ecological orientation of health promotion. The move toward social ecology is a move towards a framework for understanding the constellation of core principles and theories and the interrelationship and dynamic interplay between individual, community and organisational analytic levels (Stokols 1996).

Although overlapping with previous authors, most obviously in his integration of the behaviour-change and lifestyle modification approach, Stokols goes much further in highlighting the theoretical and research constructs associated with:

- behaviour change
- environmental enhancement
- social ecology.

He also presents in table format a summary of these in relation to health (and illness) determinants and focus and types of health promotion intervention, and advances the application of middle-range theories to health problems and interventions based on qualitative analysis of contextual factors. The table does not include examples of outcomes but these are later developed within his six procedural guidelines for designing, implementing and evaluating community health promotion programmes. Overall, this is a thorough analysis of complex issues and theory and a comprehensive guide to social ecological health promotion based on six domains, although these overlap, that most interestingly does not expressly comprise bottom-up self/community empowerment processes.

CONCLUSION

As can be seen from the review of the general health education and health promotion frameworks in this chapter, the array of competing and co-existing theoretical constructions and terminology that have emerged over the years ostensibly suggests a broad range of practice interventions. However, irrespective of the year of publication many are but variations on a theme, cover the same theoretical terrain and reflect the same aims, methods and outcomes. In addition, their models can be accounted for by Beattie's (1991) general health promotion framework and thus by implication those of Piper and Brown (1998a) and Piper (2000, 2004, 2007a, 2007b) in relation to nursing.

The majority of the frameworks reviewed, then, are descriptive, superficial, pragmatic factor-isolating theories (see Chapter 2). They are devoid of epistemological and methodological considerations and of any reference to their ideological perspective or relationship to broader social theory and more general theoretical analysis. There is an absence of reflexivity, much of the power analysis is superficial and for the most part their models are presented in an eclectic and pluralistic but insufficiently comprehensive manner.

For Rawson (2002), many of the frameworks are about modes of service delivery and appear to have been produced to help explain a particular intervention or to outline approaches various professional groups could adopt in practice. They describe how health promotion happens rather than explore the founding values and conflicts (Jones and Naidoo 2000). Rawson (2002) contends that the volume of general frameworks has caused confusion and inhibited the theoretical growth of a subject area that is inadequately structured, built on shaky philosophical foundations and which has failed to produce a body of knowledge worthy of discipline status.

Some of the authors are excused the criticisms of theoretical shallowness in drawing on an established and accepted framework for social theory and organisational analysis. Caplan's (1993) theoretical mapping exercise (see Chapter 2) is similar in principle to Beattie in advancing that the emergent models of health promotion are empirical manifestations of quintessential theoretical positions and structures. The problem is that in grafting Burrell and Morgan's (1979) metatheoretical framework onto health promotion, and in translating each of the social theory paradigms into models of health promotion, his framework is more tentative and lacks the clarity, precision and potential for detailed application of Beattie.

Other exceptions include, for example, French and Adams (1986) but they exclude legislative models, the highly informed and influential Tones (1981, 1986) and his co-authored work (Tones *et al.* 1990; Tones and Tilford 1994, 2001; Tones and Green 2004), Caraher (1994b) and the ecologists. The ecologists are comprehensive in their construction and classification of models of health promotion and in their integrative person–behaviour–environment ideology, but their theorising is of a technical and pragmatic nature and is thus more narrowly focused than Beattie (1991). Indeed, in contrast to Beattie (1991), none of the authors exposes the founding theoretical assumptions of their work with such detail and clarity or have the symmetry of the architecture of his framework. This leaves Beattie's (1991) framework and its nursing-specific derivatives (Piper and Brown 1998a, Piper 2000, 2004, 2007a, 2007b) in pole position. Chapter 4 poses the final test by presenting and reviewing health education and health promotion frameworks used by nurses, or those constructed for or by nurses, which can be used as another benchmark against which Beattie's (1991) and thus Piper and Brown's (1998a) and Piper's (2000, 2004, 2007a, 2007b) work can be measured.

LEARNING TRIGGERS

Having read Chapter 3, complete the learning triggers below to reinforce your understanding of the concepts that have been discussed:

- Identify whether the general health promotion frameworks reviewed are factor-isolating or factor-relating theories (these concepts are explained in Chapter 2).
- Identify in what ways the general health promotion frameworks reviewed illuminate their ideological perspectives, relationship to wider social theory and more general theoretical analysis.
- Identify in what ways the general health promotion frameworks reviewed undertake a power analysis in relation to the models they enumerate and the relationship between the health promoter (i.e. nurse) and the client/patient.
- Identify the weaknesses of the general health promotion frameworks reviewed in relation to the Beattie (1991) (see Chapter 2) and thus the Piper and Brown (1998a) and Piper (2000, 2004, 2007a, 2007b) frameworks.

HEALTH EDUCATION AND HEALTH PROMOTION

4

NURSING FRAMEWORKS AND PRACTICE

INTRODUCTION

Health education and health promotion might be espoused as a fundamental part of nursing, but Piper (2007b) notes that the extensive range of literature on health education and health promotion readily accessible in any nursing library or online is mostly of a pragmatic nature and concerned with 'doing'. Piper (2007b) highlights that fundamental questions about purpose, fit with practice and detailed analysis of the different frameworks and models and their relevance for nursing, particularly in relation to specialist areas of practice, remain an underdeveloped area. Scrutiny and clarification of their philosophical foundations, their relationship to wider social theory and description of how to operationalise them were similarly found wanting.

Research on the knowledge, understanding and health education/ promotion practice of nurses in hospitals is also limited (Latter 1993; Caraher 1994b; Maidwell 1996; Twinn and Lee 1997; Whitehead 1999a; Latter 2001; Piper 2004; Cross 2005). It would seem there has been less emphasis placed on health education and promotion here than in the community (Latter 1993; Whitehead 1999a; Piper 2004; Cross 2005).

Hence this chapter, based on aspects of the work of Piper (2004), reviews the frameworks and models developed or advanced for use by nurses by following the same processes and organisational format as Chapter 3. As before, the review includes frameworks that include two or more models of health education/promotion but differs in that it also refers to examples of sole models of practice, including from psychology, to help illustrate the breadth of the debate and range of issues that nursing seeks to address.

It also reviews a small number of mostly UK studies undertaken and theory-focused articles written on health education and health promotion and nursing. It is important to stress that this is not a systematic review but, as with Chapter 3, an attempt to highlight the tenor, character and emphasis of the debate via selected publications and to help illustrate the status afforded health education and health promotion theory by nursing. In further helping to gain an under-standing of the nature of health education/promotion in nursing and related theorising, this chapter will help the reader to consider the potential of specific nursing frameworks to challenge Beattie (1991), Piper and Brown (1998a) and Piper (2000, 2004, 2007a, 2007b) and the framework of the book advanced in Chapter 5.

The historical and contextual influences of these frameworks and models are the same for the UK authors cited in the 1980s, and whose later work is a continuation of the same themes, as those of Chapter 3. This is also true for some of the later authors. For example, Cork (1990) and Kuss *et al.* (1997) draw on the work of the WHO (1984) but this is less explicit in the work of others and absent in some such as Pender (1996) and Wu and Pender (2005) whose focus is limited to psychology. As with previous chapters, the variation in the use of the terms health education and health promotion reflect the way the different writers use them.

LEARNING OUTCOMES

By reading this chapter, and completing the learning triggers at the end, the reader should have a better conceptual grasp of theory and research in relation to:

* health education and health promotion frameworks and models and nursing;
* health education, health promotion and nursing practice;
* health promotion and Project 2000-educated nurses;
* thematically related literature on health promotion in hospitals and nursing.

THEORY

HEALTH EDUCATION AND HEALTH PROMOTION FRAMEWORKS AND NURSING

Cork (1990)

Cork describes and translates into pragmatic approaches for community nursing the WHO (1984) aims of:

- advocacy
- enabling
- mediation

and their framework for health promotion. Advocacy for health aims to make political, economic, social, cultural, behavioural and biological factors favourable through collecting and presenting individual and community data and developing skills in individual and community advocacy. The enabling approach aims to enhance health potential and reduce health status inequality through increasing knowledge and understanding on health matters, developing individual coping strategies, improving access to health and creating supportive environments.

Mediation health promotion takes place between differing interests in society with the aim of getting co-ordinated action to improve health by the government, the public sector, non-statutory organisations, industry and the media. This is achieved by community nurses identifying local health issues, influencing local and national policy by lobbying, presenting evidence, participating in policy formation on working parties and using the influence of their trade unions and professional organisations.

Each approach has four strands addressing individual and collective health promotion issues. Cork (1990) rightly stresses the need to intervene on all levels and move beyond the individual lifestyle and behaviour-change approaches to health promotion and embrace collaborative working in the community. Nevertheless, there is duplication and a methodological blurring between and within the approaches and no explicit analysis of power relationships. Cork also omits to say how community nurses can change the political climate to allow them to shift their practice into the socio-political arena at the expense of their traditional role.

Foster and Mayall (1990)

An investigation of mothers' and health visitors' views on good child health care provides the backdrop for Foster and Mayall's (1990) four (three of which are untitled) models of health education. These are sketched out in brief within the parameters of who sets the agenda, methods and individualistic or structural interventions. Their framework includes the ubiquitous top-down and health educator-led traditional model, which predetermines the desired health-related behaviour(s) of the client and aims to achieve client compliance through overt and covert methods. Their second model also aims for behaviour change but through two-way dialogue and an active definition of problems by the learner.

Models three and four focus on structural issues and are also divided by their method of intervention. The third model, like the first, has the agenda set by the educator but here the focus is on circumstances and a change in behaviour consistent with environmental change, such as physical improvements to where they live or increased welfare benefits. The fourth model pursues the same outcomes but from a perspective of professional–client dialogue and shared identification of need.

The outcomes of their small-scale study are particularly interesting (but perhaps unsurprising) in relation to expressed preference for ways of working. Health visitors preferred top-down, individualistic health education interventions aimed at the health-related behaviour of the client complying with the predetermined professional agenda. The mothers, whose views were polarised from those of the health visitors, preferred a dialogue with their own priorities as the starting point.

Caraher (1994b)

Caraher's work contains four approaches to health promotion that derive from a sociological analysis of the influences professional and organisational processes have on health promotion in institutional settings. Caraher identifies community nurses historically with health promotion and hospital nurses with care and cure. He contends that the latter fail to make the link between the relevance of health promotion and diseased hospitalised patients and thus engage in minimal intervention. Caraher supports this contention by reference to the findings of a small-scale survey he undertook on student nurses.

The location of power and control are central to his analysis, and Caraher's contention is that the value accorded health promotion in hospital is related to its perceived usefulness and benefit to the smooth running and administration of the hospital. Success is measured by maintenance of hierarchies, reduced duration of in-patient stay, reduced need for pain relief and financial savings and is inextricably linked to patient compliance. Health promotion practice is most likely to fall within the authoritative guidance model that maximises the professional power exercised by nurses. Here, nurse control and responsibility is high and patient control and responsibility is low (Caraher 1994b).

Caraher advocates the use of three of the approaches in his framework in a sequenced fashion, along a continuum of patient dependence to independence, to meet the needs of the hospital and the nurse–patient relationship. Although critical of authoritative guidance, he suggests that this may be an appropriate starting point in response to initial patient uncertainty and the need for institutional control. This should then progress to active patient-participation health promotion, the most effective approach for meeting patient needs (Caraher 1994b) and ultimately to independent patient decision-making to aid preparation for patient discharge.

Sequenced health promotion omits the decision-making by default approach, although precisely what this stands for is not made clear. Indeed the aims, methods and outcomes of all the approaches could be embellished further to assist in the use and application to practice of a most interesting theoretical construction that explicitly maps the potential power dynamics of the nurse–patient health promotion relationship. Answers as to how established institutional power structures can be challenged also need to be offered.

Davis (1995)

Davis explicitly generates a model for health promotion both from her qualitative findings and review of the literature. Davis describes the model as integrating the patient, the nurse, rehabilitation, health education and health promotion and founded on the principles of empowerment. The associated elements of the latter are to do with decision-making and goal planning, and patient, family and nurse partnership with the patient as co-manager of their care and the nurse adopting the role of advocate.

The premise for the model is that the rehabilitation patient is considered healthy, which is interesting given that the patients are in hospital and are impaired as a result of disease, and that health promotion and the process of rehabilitation are concerned with wellness. Davis cites the model as a framework for practice to improve both nursing care and patient empowerment and thus self-esteem in neurological rehabilitation, but contends that the model is transferable to other rehabilitation settings. Davis is to be applauded as one of the few nursing authors to have constructed a model and as such makes a valuable contribution to the debate. However, the model is only sketched out and its theory base, ideological connotations, mode of application and fine detail need developing.

Kemm and Close (1995)

Kemm and Close provide an embellished list of health promotion activities and briefly sketch out three models of health promotion for undergraduate students of nursing and health. The tenor of knowledge–attitude–behaviour (KAB) is that of medical/behaviour change outlined by various authors in Chapter 3, and their empowerment and community action models likewise offer nothing new.

Doty (1996)

Doty reviews the knowledge required by advanced practice nurses (APN) in the promotion of rural family health. He concludes that exposure to conceptual frameworks at the complementary micro (conservative) and macro (broad-based) levels and an understanding of how they affect APN practice is fundamental to an understanding of health problems and health promotion. The conservative theoretical approaches of Doty's two-model framework endorse the use of theories of psychology to explain and manipulate individuals' attitudes and perceptions toward health, disease, health care provision and health-related behaviour but do not take account of socio-economic determinants. Broad-based theoretical approaches focus on APNs empowering patients to improve social and community health and prevent community disequilibrium. They acknowledge the social, economic and political influences on health and the need for social reform but do not go so far as to advocate structural change.

Pender (1996), Wu and Pender (2005)

The Health Promotion Model (HPM) (Pender 1996) and the Revised Health Promotion Model (RHPM) as tested by Wu and Pender (2005) are theoretical constructions for use in nursing practice that Pender says have been theory tested on a number of occasions and subsequently modified. The HPM and RHPM integrate established psychology theories of health behaviour with nursing perspectives. When seen schematically, they are clearly reminiscent of models from the former discipline such as the Health Belief Model (HBM). Syred

(1981) advanced this for health education practice by hospital nurses as a way of redressing an abdication of the role, as did Roden (2004), in a modified form, for health promotion with young families. As with psychology theories and models of human behaviour such as the HBM, the purpose of the HPM and RHPM are to explain and predict health- and illness-related behaviour. The HPM excludes fear and threat as motivators and acknowledges the influence on lifestyle of the environment with the RHPM extending this to gender and socio-economic factors.

The HPM and RHPM are based on assumptions that people make rational goal-directed decisions and actively regulate their own health-related behaviour and lifestyle. They assume that individuals value personal growth and that there are a range of precursors, processes and stages to change that can be influenced. These include, for example, dissatisfaction with their prevailing situation, the likely and desired outcomes of health-related behaviour change, self-efficacy and vicarious learning. The role of the nurse is to understand the multidimensional character of health-related behaviour, the psychological variables that influence change and use the model to help patients attain positive health outcomes. This is achieved through shaping behaviour by emphasising the positive benefits of lifestyle modification, teaching patients how to overcome barriers to change, engendering high levels of self-efficacy and reinforcing change through giving positive feedback.

The HPM, RHPM and HBM offer valuable insight into the motivation behind health-related behaviour and can thus make a valuable contribution to nursing practice, but they reflect the narrow agenda of the top-down nurse as behaviour change agent (Chapter 6) and are thus limited in focus. Hence, if the HPM, RHPM or HBM are used in isolation by nurses to manipulate and direct patients toward nurse-determined health promotion outcomes, then strategic, patient control and empowerment-based outcomes will be overlooked. In addition, for Whitehead (2005b) the use of the term health promotion does not reflect contemporary usage and the narrow focus of the HPM and RHPM (and thus Roden's (2004) revised HBM) are actually consistent with health education.

Kuss *et al.* (1997)

There is also a degree of conceptual murkiness in Kuss *et al.*'s (1997) public health nursing (PHN) model. The new-age style model represented as a flowering tree was developed to define roles and practice. There are seven parts to the flowering tree model, which symbolise nine explicit and four implicit PHN concepts. One of the nine concepts has the four public health outcomes of

- promotion
- protection
- prevention
- access

which are the foliage of the tree and the product of multidisciplinary, multi-sector and community alliances whose intervention may go beyond the outcomes.

The WHO (1984) definition of health promotion as a process of increasing control over health determinants by individuals and communities, partly through political action, is quoted. Health education mobilises health- and social-service providers and service users. Examples of topics for health promotion intervention are physical activity and fitness and education programmes on nutrition, substance misuse, sexuality and parenting. Whitehead (2006) would equate these examples with health education rather than health promotion and would criticise the authors accordingly.

Health protection promotes health through legislative and statutory public health interventions on such issues as air and water quality and sanitation. Prevention includes primary, secondary and tertiary interventions as discussed in Chapter 1, and access is simply appropriate and timely use of health services. Many would view protection, prevention and access as part of the wider contemporary health promotion agenda and Kuss *et al.*'s conceptually vague discussion lacks cohesion and omits to develop individual or community empowerment models of health promotion. This is despite the latter being cited as one of the key concepts defining PHN practice.

Piper and Brown (1998a) and Piper (2000)

Piper and Brown apply a modified version of Beattie's (1991) framework of health promotion models (see Chapter 2) to nursing, which they rename as:

- patient information model;
- patient empowerment model;
- structural change model;
- collective action model.

Piper and Brown argue that the social determinants of health and health-related behaviour need to be considered by nurses as a powerful factor in the formation of lifestyles. Therefore, any health promotion strategy should employ, to varying degrees, all four of the models in the framework to form a comprehensive repertoire of nursing health promotion interventions. However, they only translate into practice the aims, methodologies and outcomes of the two 'polarised' models of health education (see Chapter 1 for differentiation between health education and health promotion) they contend are most likely to be operationalised by nurses in clinical settings. Piper (2000) adapted slightly the Piper and Brown (1998a) framework and relabelled the latter two models as strategy and policy development model, and patient action model respectively when mapping health promotion activity at institutional and clinical levels, but only outlines superficially the framework and its models.

Smith and Cusack (2000)

Smith and Cusack highlight the use of the five strategies of the *Ottawa Charter* for health promotion (see Chapter 1) specifically as a framework for managing drug and alcohol issues in Australia in line with the national context. Thus, its potential for use beyond this specialist area of practice is not considered, there is no wider debate re frameworks and models of health promotion or detailed analysis of the strategies of the framework. The focus is on testing the depth of nurses' knowledge of the charter and the challenges of applying it to practice. Although the strategies in relation to the latter are only addressed superficially the authors conclude that the *Ottawa Charter* has the potential to be strengthened and thus developed as a useful framework for alcohol- and drug-related nursing practice.

Whitehead (2001a, 2001b) and related work

Whitehead's (2001b) broad, erudite contribution to the debate includes a cognitive behavioural model for health education practice in nursing based on established theories of psychology, with Gonser and McGuiness (2001) also drawing on the latter. They include Pender's HPM to reinforce social learning theory, cognitive theory and the health belief model when advancing the theory base of health promotion for acute care nurse practitioners. There is nothing to be gained by a detailed examination of the work of these authors here as, suffice to say, the strengths and limitations of Pender's work are of the same order for Whitehead (2001b) and Gonser and McGuiness' advocacy of the use of theories and models of psychology as a basis for changing the health trajectory of patients.

In addition, Whitehead's (2001a) stage-planning programme model for health promotion practice is a comprehensive planning model. In integrating competing perspectives it guides the planning and process of individual- and collective-action nursing intervention. It is, however, primarily an iconic (Rawson and Grigg 1988; Rawson 1990) or technical (Tones and Tilford 2001) model (see Chapter 2).

Thomson's (1998) planning compass for health promotion in the nursing curriculum and Skybo and Polivka's (2006) highly specific, pragmatic model for preventing childhood violence combining public health, collaborative and psychosocial approaches with primary, secondary and tertiary prevention also fit into this category. The same can be said of the educational career youth development model (Tabi 2002) developed for preventing teenage pregnancy. This inclusive model takes account of a range of variables within five elements from social learning theory and thus an individual action perspective and with a predetermined, i.e. top-down, agenda.

Berg and Sarvimäki (2003)

Berg and Sarvimäki are concerned with the preliminary aspects of a potential holistic-existential health promotion framework. They seek to make explicit its philosophical foundation as they find this so often absent in related nursing work and call for health promotion in nursing to be reconceptualised and distanced from the medical model. The holistic-existential approach is essentially an individual action, person-centred model of health promotion based on humanism, holism, personal autonomy and a bottom up emphasis with nurse–patient dialogue as central to the process and fits with the nurse as empowerment facilitator agenda in Chapter 7 herein.

Kiger (2004)

Kiger's framework outlines five models of health education and their concomitant assumptions, strategy, tactics and role of the practitioner although these are not developed explicitly in relation to nursing. It is a revised version of the work of Coutts and Hardy (1985). For Kiger the models co-exist, overlap, are complementary, need not operate in isolation and should be applied to practice in response to circumstance and need.

The medical and educational models are as for the approaches of previous authors described in Chapter 3 (for example, Ewles and Simnett 2003). The political approach equates with societal change and community development with the client-directed approaches of Ewles and Simnett (2003) and the empowerment approach of Naidoo and Wills (2000). The introduction of the ostensibly different media (propaganda) model is something of a red herring. It merely represents a narrower version of the behaviour-change approaches of the other authors and Kiger creates something of a false dichotomy between this and her version of the medical model as they both seem to represent variations on a theme.

Piper (2004, 2005, 2007a, 2007b)

Piper (2004) employed qualitative theory-testing techniques and research methodology to test the degree of fit between Beattie's (1991) health promotion framework and fieldwork findings. Although the degree of fit between these and thus the Piper and Brown (1998) and Piper (2000) frameworks were not absolute in all cases, the pragmatic and conceptual links identified were strong enough to allow the revised framework to be tentatively advanced for consideration for nursing health-promotion practice. Reconfiguring the framework in this way and reconceptualising the existing theory via theory derivation and synthesis (see Chapter 5) and by using the themes and deviant/paradigm case findings from the fieldwork to rename the models gave new meaning to phenomena from a nursing perspective. Constructive theorising was also used to reconceptualise and apply the framework to midwifery in the same way (Piper 2005).

Piper (2004) acknowledges that the qualitative findings of the small-scale theory testing study are not generalisable and that the theory–practice relationship and the durability and transferability of the derived work requires additional research/theory testing. This prompted further revision of the framework (Piper 2007a, 2007b) to more clearly articulate the knowledge and power base of the models of practice and their intertwined relationships in relation to individual and macro/micro patient population foci of intervention. This forms the template of the framework of the book, which is more fully developed in Chapter 5 with each model discussed in full in subsequent chapters to help nurses identify, chart and plan clinically focused interventions and strategic, organisational and patient-led processes.

93

In theory, the size of the profession and interpersonal nature of nursing means that it is ideally placed to lead health promotion intervention in a variety of settings in general (Whitehead 2005a) and in the hospital setting in particular (Latter 2001). In practice this is not happening and a different mindset (Whitehead 2005a) and more training (Casey 2007; Kelly and Abraham 2007), resources and support from management (Kelly and Abraham 2007) together with the use of action research (Casey 2007) might help nursing to meet this opportunity.

Over the years the limited number of studies undertaken on health promotion and nursing, albeit generally with small sample sizes, reveals a narrow range of practice. The only major UK study of this type was a Department of Health-sponsored national investigation into nurses' perceptions of health education and the extent to which health education is incorporated into nursing practice in acute settings (Macleod Clark *et al.* 1991; Latter *et al.* 1992). Postal questionnaires were sent to senior nurses who were asked to identify acute wards engaged in health education within the five predetermined categories of:

- patient education;
- information giving;
- healthy lifestyle advice;
- facilitating patient participation in care;
- facilitating family participation in care.

The differences between the categories in terms of what each represents precisely were not outlined and whether these differences were explained to the respondents is not made clear. The authors found that health education played a part in nursing practice in acute settings. The emphasis was on intervention within the first three categories rather than on encouraging patient and family participation in care.

Wilson-Barnett and Latter (1993), Piper (2004), Casey (2007), Whitehead *et al.* (2007) and Kelly and Abraham (2007) support the above findings, which emphasise the traditional patient education and information-giving aspects of practice in the hospital setting. For Wilson-Barnett and Latter (1993) and Casey (2007) health education/ promotion did not take account of more contemporary and wider aspects of intervention such as collaboration, participation and empowerment. Information-giving was largely focused on disease, orientation to the clinical setting, realistic expectations regarding treatment and preoperative information. Some of the information given was by way of reacting to patients' questions, but even when asked some nurses did not respond to cues or questions (Wilson-Barnett and Latter 1993).

Much of this is consistent with the findings of Gott and O'Brien (1990a), Maidwell (1996) and Twinn and Lee (1997) in reflecting a medical, and thus didactic and authoritarian, model of nurse–patient interaction. Twinn and Lee (1997) advance that nurses limit their definition of health education to patient information. Activity relating to this definition ranges from promoting health and disease prevention, to simply patient orientation to the clinical setting, but the emphasis is on the patient's disease and medical treatment. Health education in acute care is a minimal feature of practice, tends to occur during admission or around the time of discharge and does not extend to collaborating with patients or encouraging their participation in care.

However, Piper (2004, 2007a) reports that although information-giving was largely informal, unplanned, reactive, submerged in the milieu of practice and often of a conversational nature, it did fit with aspects of individual and group empowerment and strategic objectives. Whiting (2001) also noted a wider health promotion agenda in her small-scale qualitative study with children's nurses (three community and three hospital-based) and her findings espouse a sensitive and intuitive approach to families, role modelling, teamwork, patient participation and commitment.

McBride's (1994) exploration of the attitudes, beliefs and health promotion practices of nurses in acute-care settings in two hospitals presented an interesting paradox. Nurses reported that they were keen to undertake health promotion but that they lacked the time and training to be effective. In addition, when patients specifically asked for lifestyle advice nurses often failed to respond and thus meet a patient identified need, even though some nurses perceived a strong link between lifestyle and advice. Intervention in general was found to be haphazard, generally unevaluated and there was an absence of coherent health promotion strategies. McBride (1995) has subsequently sought to provide a solution to this by writing a step-by-step instruction handbook for nurses on how to undertake practical health promotion in hospital.

Maidwell's (1996) focus was slightly narrower in researching the health promotion practice of nurses working in surgical settings. She was consistent with McBride (1994) in establishing that health promotion was not only part of the role, but an essential element that goes hand-in-hand with nursing care. In defining health promotion, the nurses in the study emphasised disease prevention and management, but also indicated a move toward encouraging patient participation in care, education and healthy lifestyle advice. Maidwell (1996) perceives this as promoting positive health, rather than negative health where disease prevention is emphasised, although in reality it is still located in the medical model. Particular emphasis was given to the discharge interview as a time for health promotion.

Berland *et al.* (1995) also examined the knowledge, attitudes and health promotion practice of acute-care nurses. Health promotion was seen as an integral part of care and included discharge planning, empowerment, caring for families and normalising life for hospitalised patients, but much of this practice was not labelled as health promotion. Acute-care nurses were also identified as an under-utilised health promotion resource.

Jones (1993) used the five categories and raw data of Macleod Clark *et al.* (1991) to draw conclusions about opportunities for health education in acute settings and the associated type of nurse–patient interactions. Jones (1993) stresses that good communication is fundamental to successful health education. It assists in eliciting patient-defined needs and aids movement away from the medical model toward building nurse–patient relationships into partnerships. These could build on the existing knowledge and experiences of patients, help them develop a sense of autonomy and feel empowered to take responsibility and feel positive.

Quite how responsibility should be interpreted here is not entirely clear but it is a term more commonly associated with the medical, rather than the empowerment model of health education. Maben *et al.* (1993) identified that the way nursing care is organised influences and can be a potential barrier or facilitator of health education in acute-ward settings. She concluded that a move away from top-down nurse-led health education towards empowering patients is dependent on nurses also being empowered.

Although Piper (2007b) notes the absence of a unifying framework for classifying health promotion theory and practice in nursing both in general and in relation to emergency nursing, Cross (2005) was struck by the absence of any research into the attitudes of nurses in this specialist clinical setting. Although not generalisable due to the small sample size, Cross's (2005) research into this found a positive attitude and commitment toward health promotion by the emergency nurses in the study. The impact of socio-economic influences on health was acknowledged as were contemporary concepts such as empowerment (though not defined), but Cross nevertheless concluded that a broader understanding of health promotion is needed.

Irvine's (2005) research using the Delphi technique set out to identify the competencies required by district nurses for effective health promotion. She found a consensus among panellists of the need for a range of competencies within the categories of knowledge, attitudes and skills. Unsurprisingly, many of the competencies within the categories overlap with other aspects of practice and thus Irvine concludes that district nurses already have a sound foundation for practice. The research raises some interesting issues for nurse education and for developing the district nursing role but the work is criticised by Whitehead (2006) for the way in which the term health promotion is used as he takes the view that what is being described is health education.

Whitehead's (2006) criticism may also extend to the way Kelly and Abraham (2007) use the term health promotion when using psychology theory to investigate nurses' perceptions of their role with hospitalised patients over 65 years old, although they do acknowledge empowerment as part of health promotion. They reported that the majority of the participants had a positive attitude toward health promotion. It was considered part of the nursing role and participants felt able and willing to fulfil this aspect of practice although felt that for some patients it was inappropriate, was more difficult to achieve with those over 75 and that practice was constrained by organisational barriers.

HEALTH EDUCATION AND HEALTH PROMOTION WITHIN A REHABILITATION SETTING

Information-giving was the predominant form of intervention, with teaching described as health education by 10 out of the 18 nurses working in a neurological rehabilitation setting (Davis 1995). Of the participants, 13 saw health education as synonymous with the rehabilitation role of nurses, with the key aims of teaching patients both how to cope with the changes induced by their illness and how to exercise informed choice. The emphasis was on encouraging patients to be involved in their own rehabilitation programme.

Davis (1995) did endeavour to unpack the nurses' perceptions of the difference between health education and health promotion and the latter was associated with health education plus the addition of wider environmental and political issues. Later in the article health promotion is also linked to raising awareness, promoting self-esteem and being an effective role model. The waters are slightly muddied by Davis who goes on to say that there was a consensus that health promotion and rehabilitation were integrated, whereas initially the term health education had been used to describe this unity. From this work Davis (1995) constructed the model for health promotion outlined earlier in this chapter.

HEALTH PROMOTION AND PROJECT 2000-EDUCATED NURSES

The level of understanding and the health promotion role of Project 2000-educated nurses features in the literature (Macleod Clark and Maben 1998; McDonald 1998). Macleod Clark and Maben (1998) present the findings from a large-scale two-centre case study for the English National Board for Nursing, Midwifery and Health Visiting. They found that although participants felt that there was a difference between health education and health promotion there was some conceptual confusion over their defining characteristics. This confusion extended to a sophisticated understanding of philosophy underpinning various forms of health gain and of the need for a broader range of interventions to achieve this outcome, such as holism and empowerment, but a failure to link these to health promotion and related intervention.

Thus, descriptions of health promotion by students emphasised top-down, individual health-related behaviour and lifestyle approaches. This narrow focus echoes the earlier biomedical emphasis of philosophy of health and health promotion in the educational curriculum and its integration in four nurse-education institutions in England in the predominantly qualitative study of Smith *et al.* (1995a, 1995b).

Conversely, the small study by McDonald (1998) on nurses working in a hospital setting found that their perceptions of health promotion include, but also go beyond, traditional information-giving and patient teaching. The nurses perceived health promotion to include modes of practice that embrace supporting and encouraging patients in their decision-making, negotiating and collaborating over patient need, involving patients and their significant others in care management, advocacy and empowerment. They also acknowledged the psycho-social determinants of health. Similarly, Hills (1998) conducted a qualitative study of the experiences of 24 student nurses of health promotion in hospital nursing practice. She cites the primacy given to patients as people, and the nurse–patient relationship, a person-centred approach to practice, empowerment, patient participation and nurse–patient partnership and an awareness of the social context of the patient's life as evidence of nursing interventions with a clear health promotion perspective.

In a similar vein, Mitchenson (1995) compared the attitudes and beliefs on health education and health promotion held by student nurses that were educated in a traditional way with those that undertook a Project 2000 course. Ward (1997) also explored this territory with similar cohorts and looked at student nurses' perceptions of health promotion and perceptions of the role of the nurse as a health promoter.

In the main, Mitchenson found enthusiasm for the health promotion aspect of the nurse's role that was seen as an important part of practice. There was agreement that health promotion involved modifying unhealthy behaviour and that the nurse is dominant in the process. Examples of where there were disagreements included more emphasis given to psychosocial wellbeing, less tolerance of circumstances impeding health promotion, but paradoxically also a greater tendency to coercion by Project 2000 students. Another difference was that traditionally trained nurses felt that there was insufficient time to practise health promotion. Although some in Holt and Warne's (2007) study concur with this, the student nurses also reported a lack of opportunity. The health promotion role of nurses was recognised but the problem with putting theory into practice was attributed to poor role modelling by qualified nurses, its perceived low priority and relevance and the way in which the subject was taught.

Overall, Ward (1997) found the perceptions of health promotion practice narrow, with conceptual confusion among students when asked to explain the difference between health promotion and nursing. Although the theory base of Project 2000 students was much stronger than those conventionally trained, even though the latter actually placed more value on that aspect of the nurse's role, the general findings of Ward (1997) concur with those of the authors above. Health promotion was predominantly seen as information-giving and lifestyle and risk factor advice rather than about more empowering-type strategies, and the responses of the students indicated an adherence to hospital routines.

THEMATICALLY RELATED LITERATURE ON HEALTH PROMOTION IN HOSPITALS AND NURSING

The traditional position adopted by authors discussing the health-education and health-promotion role of hospital nurses was to emphasise the need to influence, and help patients modify, health beliefs (Syred 1981) and lifestyle together with extolling the virtues of disease-related teaching (Flynn and Giffin 1984). More contemporary writing considering the potential for health promotion practice in hospital settings has broadened the debate.

For Latter (2001), historically health promotion by hospital nurses was limited to traditional, top-down health education interventions that fit with the nurse as behaviour change agent (see Chapter 6). Examples include preparing patients for surgery, which includes ensuring that they are well-informed about the procedure and is known to reduce anxiety and expedite recovery. However, this traditional medical-model stance, and the cure- and treatment-based orientation of nursing care that has concomitant expectations of patient passivity and compliance, clashes with the emergent values and concepts central to health promotion of empowerment, public participation and partnership working. Latter (2001) calls for changes to the traditional patterns of health promotion practice of nurses. Nursing needs to embrace issues to do with patient self-efficacy and patient-centred approaches and to reject any form of coercion. Further to this, Latter advocates that hospital nurses develop a broader, collaborative health promotion role and address the wider barriers to patient health promotion.

Latter (2001) posits that hospital nurses could engage in critical consciousness raising by educating patients about health determinants and the politics of health to catalyse community action for change. More grounded suggestions include liaison with other professional groups, community agencies, acting as key agents of influence for health promotion strategic and policy development within hospitals, identifying trends in hospital admission and contributing their findings to local health-care needs assessment. Latter also contends that nurses can facilitate the setting up of self-help groups for patients and carers with similar experiences and traumas and offer continued support to these forums.

Whitehead (1999a) summarises the literature considering the nature of health promotion in acute and community settings. Despite health and social policy, legislative and advisory bodies and the nursing literature pushing for the development of health promotion in hospital nursing, the status quo predominates. He points to the enormity of the task ahead in moving hospital nurses away from current traditional interventions to more contemporary ones and in developing a clear way forward for practice. Whitehead (1999b) endeavours to point the way by applying health promotion concepts to the narrow practice setting of orthopaedic nursing and by adapting the five approaches of Ewles and Simnett (see Chapter 3 herein) to broaden the debate. He has some success with this, particularly from an individual action perspective but less so in relation to intervention for collective health gain. A more sophisticated and broader version of the former is developed later in Whitehead's writing, for example, in 2001b and 2001c. Whitehead (1999a) also takes the view that the blame for orthodox practice cannot solely be levelled at nurses as there also needs to be a shift in health service policy that makes health promotion a service priority.

CONCLUSION

Like the general health education and health promotion frameworks reviewed in Chapter 3, many of those constructed by nurses or for use in nursing are essentially descriptive and pragmatic devices or exclude wider modes of intervention. There are others that could have been considered but they are of the same ilk. The main weakness is in failing to move beyond being factor-isolating theory or to clarify the ideological assumptions that underpin the various models in the frameworks reviewed and in not taking account of wider theoretical perspectives and metatheoretical concepts. They also tend not to illustrate the points of convergence, divergence and the inherent tensions and complementary aspects of the models. As a result their focus is much narrower than Beattie (1991) and hence Piper and Brown (1998a) and Piper (2000, 2004, 2007a, 2007b).

However, although Beattie (1991), Piper and Brown (1998a) and Piper (2000, 2004, 2007a, 2007b) articulate the client/nurse–patient power relationship and make explicit the objective and subjective epistemological positions and the individual and communitarian emphasis, they contend that each of the models is mutually exclusive. Chapter 5 further develops these and the Piper (2007a, 2007b) frameworks specifically for nursing, but differs in containing three models of health promotion that are not advanced as mutually exclusive or entirely discrete but as overlapping and where one model can help achieve the outcomes of another.

From the published theorising and research reviewed on health education, health promotion and nursing it is apparent that a tension exists between the breadth of the interventions in some of the frameworks and models and the practice of hospital nurses. This is accompanied by something of a predilection in some quarters for models inspired by psychology. These factors translate into an orientation toward information-giving and health/disease-related learning for patients. This individual action perspective has an important role to play when assisting patients in gaining knowledge and developing an understanding about their disease, its management and the contribution they can make toward maximising associated health gain. The problem is that these interventions emphasise patient compliance and action on health/disease-related behaviour within the boundaries determined by nurses, the institutions they represent and the disease process itself. They reinforce the power and control nurses exercise over patients (Caraher 1994b) and represent only a partial response to health promotion needs.

Attributing lifestyle choices and health-related behaviour as the primary determinants of health minimises the impact of social and material variables. However, as Freudenberg (1984/5) contends, health promotion activity mirrors the social forces that support it and in reflecting a traditional medical-model explanation of health nurses are reflecting the socio-political, ideological and organisational context of their practice.

LEARNING TRIGGERS

Having read Chapter 4, complete the learning triggers below to reinforce your understanding of the concepts that have been discussed:

- Identify whether the nursing health education and health promotion models and frameworks reviewed are factor-isolating or factor-relating theories (these concepts are explained in Chapter 2).
- Identify in what ways the nursing health promotion models and frameworks reviewed illuminate their ideological perspectives, relationship to wider social theory and more general theoretical analysis.
- Identify in what ways the nursing health promotion models and frameworks reviewed undertake a power analysis in relation to the models they enumerate and the relationship between the nurse and the client/patient.
- Identify the weaknesses of the nursing models and health promotion frameworks reviewed in relation to the Beattie (1991) (see Chapter 2) and thus Piper and Brown (1998a), Piper (2000) and Piper (2004, 2007a, 2007b) frameworks.
- Summarise the main findings of the research into health education, health promotion and nursing practice.
- Summarise the main findings of the research into health promotion and Project 2000-educated nurses.
- Summarise the discussion on the thematically related literature on health promotion in hospitals and nursing.

THEORY

HEALTH PROMOTION FRAMEWORK FOR NURSING PRACTICE

5

INTRODUCTION

The rationale for this chapter and, indeed, this book is the absence of a consensus over a unifying framework for classifying health promotion theory and practice in nursing and the need to debate between frameworks (Rawson 2002). What follows is a detailed explanation of the framework synthesised for nursing from Beattie's (1991, 1993), Piper and Brown's (1998a) and Piper's (2000, 2004, 2007a, 2007b) work and qualitative fieldwork findings (Piper 2004) designed to help address further this theoretical gap. This is accompanied by a discussion on health promotion models evaluation and a historical overview of the debate surrounding borrowing theory and theory development, derivation and synthesis for nursing and the application of the latter herein. Thus, this chapter discusses how the framework of the book was generated through inductive research and theorising together with its structure, the relationship between its inherent models and why it is fit for purpose. In addition, it explores the relationship between the health promotion models (the nurse as behaviour change agent, the nurse as empowerment facilitator, the nurse as strategic practitioner) within the framework and nursing practice, with subsequent chapters dedicated to each model.

INDUCTIVE HEALTH PROMOTION FRAMEWORK DEVELOPMENT

In an effort to help develop a dedicated and integrated health promotion framework for nursing that specifically translates into practice the methodologies and outcomes of a repertoire of approaches that can be operationalised in various settings, top-down theorising and an inductive, i.e. bottom-up, perspective generated from qualitative research findings were combined. The latter derives from research into the meanings hospital nurses gave to health promotion and testing the degree of fit between the findings and existing theory (Piper 2004, 2007a, 2008).

Piper (2004) collected qualitative data by individual and focus group interviews and the Critical Incident Technique (CIT) (Flanagan 1954). The latter particularly suited the theoretical focus of the research in facilitating the exploration and clarification of the language and meaning of health promotion through discussion and the sharing of perceptions and reactions to the contribution of others (Stewart and Shamdasani 1990; Carey 1994; Kitzinger 1995). However, it is acknowledged that the use of focus groups allows only relatively shallow data to be collected as the number of participants reduces the opportunity for individual contributions. This is at the expense of the depth of understanding that can be gleaned from other qualitative data collection methods. The power of group dynamics – the voices of the dominant – hierarchy and the associated issues of power and control are also potential limitations.

The individual/focus group interviews were partially structured using an interview guide broadly outlining the concepts (Carey 1994) to be explored to ensure consistency and a systematic approach (Patton 1990; May 1991; Holloway and Wheeler 1996) while allowing latitude for the participants' answers (Streubert and Carpenter 1999). The interview guide derived from the framework of quality indicators of the Society of Health Education and Health Promotion Specialists (Totten 1992). The framework is for measuring and monitoring the input, process and outcomes of health promotion and to help clarify the operational targets of different stages of intervention.

The CIT is a systematic, open-ended, verbal or written process (Norman *et al.* 1992) that can be used to help develop theory in qualitative research (Woolsey 1986) and for identifying gaps in knowledge and understanding (Twelker 2003). Flanagan (1954) emphasised that the CIT is a flexible method for observing human behaviour that can be modified and adapted as required and not a rigid method of data collection. In the study (Piper 2004) eight deviant/paradigm case participants were asked to develop a significant incident from their nursing practice that they had referred to in an earlier interview with the purpose of gaining deeper insight into the participants' definitions of health education/promotion and aims, methods and outcomes of practice.

Deviant case participants were those who had an unusual or unique insight (Lincoln and Guba 1985; Miles and Huberman 1994); and paradigm cases a clinical experience that stood out and offered a new and alternative perspective and understanding of nursing (Mitre *et al.* 1998). The terms are used here to depict findings that stemmed initially from those participants that offered a broader understanding of health education/promotion in relation to their nursing practice, practice setting or client group during phase one and phase two of the data collection. Phase three of the fieldwork with the deviant/ paradigm cases was to develop these unique insights to facilitate further generalisation in analytic terms to the established theory. Data were collected from retrospective accounts using the qualitative questionnaire of Benner (1984) who developed the technique for her research into levels of expertise in nursing and by interview (Woolsey 1986; Norman *et al.* 1992).

All 32 participants worked in an acute hospital and were purposively sampled from across the clinical and management grading structure and a range of hospital settings, namely:

- acute and emergency care
- older people
- oncology
- sexual health.

The intention was to generate a range of analytical variables and to test their degree of fit with existing theory as a precursor to theory development rather than to reach a shared understanding.

The audiotaped individual and focus group interviews were transcribed, coded and analysed both by following the manual guidelines of Hycner (1985) and by use of computer-assisted qualitative data software (QSR NUD*IST Vivo) to facilitate analysis triangulation. Use of Hycner's (1985) guidelines involved:

- listening to the interviews to get a sense of the whole;
- coding all the data;
- separating units of general meaning from units of relevant meaning;
- removing extraneous data;
- grouping the units of relevant meaning;
- identifying and contextualising themes from the latter.

The fieldwork was conducted according to the University Ethics Guidelines for Research for use when undertaking research with human subjects and was approved by the appropriate Research Degree Committee.

RESEARCH THEMES AND THE HEALTH PROMOTION FRAMEWORK

In summary, the role of the nurse as informer was the central theme of the findings and of health promotion and underpinned the themes and deviant/paradigm case aspects of practice (Piper 2004). It involved the dissemination of information to individual and groups of patients and carers to increase knowledge and understanding and assist with decision-making; and to management for strategic influence and corporate decision-making.

The one-to-one interpersonal focus of the themes of the nurse as behaviour change agent and the nurse as empowerment facilitator are concerned with the health-related knowledge, attitudes and life-style of individuals based on the assumption that these are key determinants of health status. However, in operating from different positions on the power continuum, they invoke different aims, methods

THEORY

and outcomes and thus different indicators of success in terms of health gain.

The nurse as behaviour change agent is top-down and expert-directed. In line with Beattie's health persuasion techniques (see Chapter 2 herein) participants maintained a 'high social distance' (Beattie 1991: 185). They derived a power base from their professional role and knowledge of biomedical research highlighting the relationship between disease, risk factors and lifestyle. Intervention emphasised control of the latter and the risks to individuals if they fail to pursue the prescribed course of action. The focus was the unique and specific health needs of individual patients as assessed by the nurse. It was concerned with what patients can do for themselves and in their own interests to maintain and improve their health, lifestyle and quality of life and factors that put this at risk. As indicated in Chapter 1, this represents a negative conception of health as it was in the context of patient pathology/disease or injury, hospital setting and client group.

Thus, the aim of intervention is to achieve behavioural outcomes as defined by the nurse and consequently therapeutic compliance and self-management in line with these by patients. This is achieved through informing, patient teaching and awareness-raising within the context of secondary prevention and is based on the assumption that patients are free to choose their health/disease-related behaviour and lifestyle.

It is unsurprising that empowerment was a theme of the findings as it reflects the language of much of the contemporary health and social care discourse and developing consumer, advocacy (DoH 2002) and 'expert patient' (DoH 2001) culture in the NHS in the UK. The focus was more on patient control and choice, a bottom-up model of intervention and a lower 'social distance' (Beattie 1991: 185) and included the role of practitioner as advocate (Beattie 1991) and helping patients adapt positively to changes in health status.

The nurse as empowerment facilitator is about helping patients understand their predicament and to think positively; psychological support; rapport building; developing a nurse–patient partnership; configuring services around the aspirations and convenience of the patient; and promoting participation in service-user groups. It also involves helping people to be aware of what treatment options are available and exercise informed choice, have some control in relation to their illness and come to terms and cope with the constraints and disabilities it imposes. Nevertheless, this is still in relation to disease management and associated boundaries and where choice is facilitated this is within the available resources and options. As such, it represents empowerment as a technology, (Tones 2001) i.e. a technical, skills-based process involving face-to-face encounters concerned with simple pragmatic day-to-day supportive and enabling strategies. Any change in the dynamic of the nurse–patient relationship is a modification of enduring and traditional roles.

The most surprising findings were the deviant/paradigm cases including strategic practice and advocacy that described atypical interventions and enable practice to be conceptualised from a macro- and micro-population focus. The title of the nurse as strategic practitioner was advanced by one participant when discussing working at a multidisciplinary and multi-agency level and with industry for organisational, policy and operational change. It included health surveillance, liaison with the other agencies, admission avoidance and thus strategic practice at an internal operational level. It is also applied herein (the health promoting hospital in Chapter 9) to operational issues at a hospital and departmental level and reflects strategic, organisational and policy interventions, professionally assessed needs and associated aims, methods and outcomes of practice. They are 'managerialist' and 'professionalist' and maintain a hierarchy and a system of subordination with the practitioner maintaining a 'high social distance' (Beattie 1991: 187).

Advocacy focuses on intervention with a patient population on an institutional scale and interventions that are client-centred and concerned with a form of micro population empowerment. Thus, it is not about advocating for patients individual needs, helping them with decision-making, fighting on their behalf for the therapeutic interventions they wanted or resisting the pressure of health care professionals for a particular course of action. It is about collective empowerment where the nurse raises the profile, lobbies and advocates on behalf of a disempowered hospital patient population and champions their needs where they lack a strong group voice and experience marginalisation.

Deductive theorising informed by an extensive review of pertinent literature and the themes of the research were then used to reconfigure the Beattie (1991) framework. Although Piper and Brown (1998a) and Piper (2000) undertook a similar exercise their modification to reflect a nursing frame of reference was purely from a theoretical perspective, i.e. their work was not grounded in the qualitative experiences of nurses or in empirical data. However, they do clearly articulate the nurse–patient power relationship on the locus of control axis, which also makes explicit the competing objective and subjective epistemological positions and the individual and population emphasis on the focus of intervention axis.

As with Beattie (1991), Piper and Brown (1998a) maintain that each of the four models is underpinned by contrasting epistemology, ideology and methodology, and support the view that each of the models is mutually exclusive. Their structure is exactly that of Beattie (1991, 1993) but with different nomenclature, while Figure 5.1 represents a theoretical development of these frameworks and of Piper's (2004, 2007a, 2007b) work based on the outcome of research referred to herein.

As can be seen in Figure 5.1, the combination of a nurse control axis (essentially a power continuum) and a patient focus axis creates three models of health promotion. Each has unique aims, processes, impact and outcomes (examples of these are tabulated for each model respectively in Chapters 6, 7, 8 and 9) but unlike Beattie (1991), Piper and Brown (1998a) and Piper (2000, 2004, 2007a, 2007b) they are not advanced as mutually exclusive or entirely discrete as elements overlap. For example, information-giving and the role of the nurse as informer as the central theme of practice pervade all models of health promotion within the framework. The nurse as behaviour change agent and the nurse as strategic practitioner diverge on the individual/ patient population axis as the former is concerned with individual patient behavioural outcomes and the latter with indirect collective health gain via strategic, managerial/organisational interventions. However, on the nurse control axis both models reflect a top-down nurse-led mode of intervention based on an objective assessment of need and nursing goals.

In addition, one may help achieve the outcomes of the other. For example, for many years smoking has been acknowledged as a major 'risk factor' linked with many diseases, and nurses (the nurse as behaviour change agent) and other health care professionals have encouraged patients to stop on a one-to-one basis in clinical practice with varying degrees of success. Compliance is now largely achieved, at least within health care settings in the UK, by the advent of no-smoking policies in hospital and Primary Care Trusts (prior to the national ban of smoking in public places) with the former interventions helping to create a climate of opinion conducive to enabling strategic change.

Similarly, when concerned with individual patient outcomes the nurse as empowerment facilitator converges with the nurse as behaviour change agent on the patient focus axis but appears polarised on the power continuum where nurse control is reduced and subjective

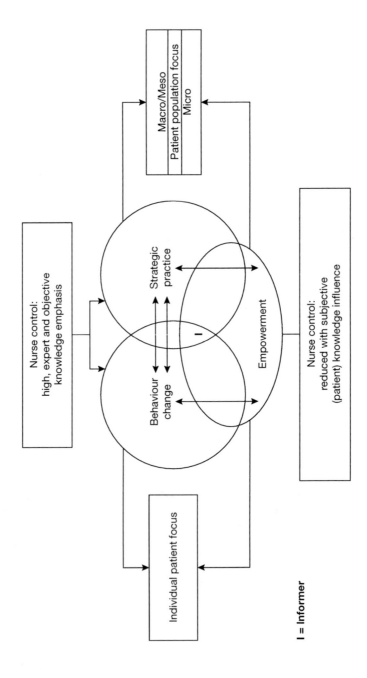

Figure 5.1 Health promotion framework

I = Informer

Nurse control: high, expert and objective knowledge emphasis

Nurse control: reduced with subjective (patient) knowledge influence

Macro/Meso
Patient population focus
Micro

Individual patient focus

Strategic practice

Behaviour change

Empowerment

patient knowledge drives a more bottom-up style of outcomes. Yet this is something of a false epistemological dichotomy. The patient can have objective knowledge and scientific understanding; and the nurse subjective knowledge, personal experience akin to that of the patient, and empathy, and the focus may be on the same health- or disease-related topics but with a different emphasis. The nurse as empowerment facilitator also converges with the nurse as strategic practitioner when the focus of intervention is at a population level while remaining divergent in terms of the locus of control. However, overlap is apparent where lobbying and the aspirations of the patient populations coincide or influence the policy decisions of nurses or there is a shared understanding of a health problem and commitment to an agenda for change.

Thus, the synthesised framework elucidates the distinctions and commonalities between various models of health promotion and illustrates diagrammatically the conceptual distinction between health education and health promotion. The nurse as behaviour change agent and the nurse as empowerment facilitator with an individual patient focus relate explicitly to health education and are ultimately orientated towards individual action interventions that can form part of a health promotion strategy. Piper and Brown (1998a) contend that any comprehensive health promotion strategy should employ all health promotion models but see clinically based nurses as involved primarily in health education. This recognises both the interpersonal nature of practice and the routine involvement in dialogue and interaction with patients, clients, relatives, groups, etc.

The nurse as strategic practitioner with a macro (societal) and meso (institutional) (Tones and Tilford 2001) population focus and the nurse as empowerment facilitator with a micro (group/community) population focus in the revised framework are thus orientated more towards health promotion than health education. They have a strategic, organisational and community focus rather than an individualistic emphasis.

It is important to note here both the problem of advancing a framework of health promotion models for, what Cormack and Reynolds (1992) describe as, a clinically heterogeneous and diverse profession caring for a range of patient/client groups, and that all models have clinical limitations. They contend that although theorists should clearly delineate the scope of their work and state its clinical application, it is for individual practitioners to evaluate and select models appropriate to their clinical situation. Cormack and Reynolds (1992) also call for models to include specific statements regarding their scope and limitations but suggest that there is an argument for saying that

nurses, rather than the theorists, should take responsibility for determining the applicability of the work to practice. In other words, it is
for the reader to judge the level of transferability of the nursing health
promotion framework and its inherent models (Figure 5.1) based on
their judgement of trustworthiness. The latter depends on the transparency of the process as revealed in earlier chapters and herein.

HEALTH PROMOTION MODELS EVALUATION

The purpose of health promotion evaluation is threefold. First, it is
to assesses how well intervention has achieved a 'valued' outcome
(WHO 1998a: 12; Tones and Green 2004: 306); was effective, i.e.
met its aims and objectives (Naidoo and Wills 2000; Tones and Tilford
2001; Whitehead 2003; Tones and Green 2004); and 'efficient' (Naidoo
and Wills 2000: 370; Whitehead 2003: 497). Efficiency refers to
how well a valued outcome was achieved relative to other interventions
(Tones and Green 2004). It also needs to be relevant ('appropriate')
'acceptable' and 'equitable' (Naidoo and Wills 2000: 370). Second,
it is to inform future planning and decision-making (Naidoo and
Wills 2000; Whitehead 2003) to make health promotion intervention
more effective (Tones and Green 2004). Third, it is part of being a
reflective practitioner (Naidoo and Wills 2000).

In simple terms, evaluation describes and appraises the health
promotion intervention of the practitioner, i.e. what was done and its
worth. It ranges from informal feedback to a more systematic review
(Naidoo and Wills 2000). However, the nurse as behaviour change
agent, the nurse as empowerment facilitator (individual and collective
action perspectives) and the nurse as strategic practitioner models
within the framework (Figure 5.1) invoke different aims, processes,
impact and outcomes and thus different indicators of success in terms
of health gain. In operating from different belief systems the models
are informed by different indicators of worth and thus different
methods of evaluation are required.

St Leger's (1999) examples of health promotion indicators that
help evaluate health promotion intervention include: biology; knowledge; attitudes; behaviour; skills; policy; environment; and partnerships.

Other examples are health literacy and community action (WHO
1998a). Health promotion evaluation, then, is not concerned solely
with behaviour change but with goals related to empowerment and
participation (Naidoo and Wills 2000) depending upon the model of
practice informing the intervention. It is also concerned not just with

outcomes but also with input (Totten 1992), process (Totten 1992; WHO 1998b; Naidoo and Wills 2000), impact (Totten 1992; Naidoo and Wills 2000) and contextual factors (WHO 1998b; Naidoo and Wills 2000). These categories create a framework for structured evaluation of health promotion intervention as defined by Totten (1992) but modified for nursing in Box 5.1.

Although there may be a tendency to focus on what Tones and Tilford (2001) and Tones and Green (2004) refer to as summative evaluation by judging the success of health promotion intervention in terms of impact and outcome after the event, process evaluation is equally valuable (WHO 1998b). Where outcome evaluation fails to shed light on why or how success was achieved (Tones 2000), process evaluation does just that (WHO 1998b; Tones and Tilford 2001) and is particularly important if the intervention needs repeating, expanding (WHO 1998b) or revising (Tones and Green 2004).

Scrutiny of process may reveal insights into key features of intervention and client perceptions and illuminate strengths and weaknesses, thus constituting a form of illuminative evaluation (Naidoo and Wills 2000; Tones and Tilford 2001). Public health nurses involved in community development projects may use the qualitative research methods of process (or formative) evaluation such as diaries, interviews and focus groups (Naidoo and Wills 2000). Although not representative or reliable in the quantitative sense, they help achieve

---

BOX 5.1 HEALTH PROMOTION EVALUATION CATEGORIES

- **Input**: nursing time, material resources, project funding.
- **Process**: i.e. what nurses and patients/clients/community members did during the intervention and how materials, resources and any project funding were used.
- **Impact**: the consequences of intervention. This is about change, i.e. behaviour, processes, procedures, facilities, environmental and organisational.
- **Outcomes**: Totten (1992) refers to this as the most problematic category as outcome targets vary by individuals and professional groups. For some, impact indicators are the most important, for others objectively measurable indicators of health status such as mortality and morbidity are what counts.

(after Totten 1992)

an understanding of the meaning members of the community gave to the experience, what they learned from it and how they have changed, and so on.

Tones and Green (2004) point out that evaluation methods are not value-free but reflect a value system and ideology. For example, as can be seen in Box 5.1, outcomes tend to be defined in terms of negative indicators of health such as mortality and morbidity. This is consistent with health promotion being associated with the health service and thus the evidence-based practice of medical model, objective, quantifiable methods of evaluation (Naidoo and Wills 2000). These fit ideologically with the nurse as behaviour change agent but are incompatible with both the individual and collective nurse as empowerment facilitator-type strategies (Naidoo and Wills 2000; Tones and Green 2004), which are as concerned with process and subjective appraisal of the worth of an intervention as they are outcome.

The traditional medical model methods of Randomised Controlled Trials and experimental research are unsuitable for trying to evaluate the interventions of the nurse as empowerment facilitator; and even for the nurse as behaviour change agent they are problematic. This is due to difficulty with isolating the effect of the health promotion activity (Naidoo and Wills 2000), the time gap between intervention and outcome, and the need for large cohort studies to demon-strate any cause and effect relationship (Tones and Tilford 2001). For example, Tones and Green (2004) refer to the problem of demon-strating the benefits of a healthy eating and exercise programme in schools when any reduction in coronary heart disease mortality and morbidity outcomes are not likely to be apparent until the pupils are well into adulthood. In addition, if the link between behaviour and outcome, i.e. mortality and morbidity, is already established then a change in the former should suffice (Tones and Tilford 2001) with data of this type justifying health promotion intervention rather than being used to indicate its effectiveness (Tones and Green 2004).

For Whitehead (2003), impact evaluation is the use of short-term, immediate feedback indicators. These can also be referred to as intermediate indicators. For some models intermediate indicators such as changes in knowledge, attitudes, beliefs and the development of skills might be more appropriate than outcome indicators (Tones 2000) and this is the contention here. Given the type of health promotion practice nurses tend to engage in, the need for short-term/immediate feedback and the lack of opportunity for large-scale quantitative experimental research and the associated practical and ideological problems with outcome evaluation, the recommendation here is for the use of impact indicators (intermediate outcomes). These, together with judging effectiveness against the aim and objectives of intervention and the process indicators should form the framework for evaluating nursing health promotion practice.

However, the nurse as behaviour change agent, the nurse as empowerment facilitator (individual and collective action perspectives) and the nurse as strategic practitioner have different socio-political and ideological foundations and modus operandi, requiring different evaluation indicators. Thus, examples of the unique aims, processes, impact (intermediate outcomes), outcomes and thus evaluatory criteria of each model are developed and illustrated in tables in Chapters 6, 7, 8 and 9.

Further to this, and under the heading of quality, the Society of Health Education and Health Promotion Specialists outline a code of practice, i.e. 'principles of good practice in health promotion' (Totten 1992: 6.4). Indicators of quality health promotion intervention adapted for nursing are:

- patient/client participation;
- promoting patient/client positive self-esteem, autonomy and choice;
- sensitivity to the socio-political determinants of health;
- ensuring the accuracy of health information;
- ensuring that health promotion nursing practice is based on up-to-date knowledge of methodologies and effectiveness.

HEALTH PROMOTION THEORY DERIVATION FOR NURSING

Chapter 2 advanced Beattie's (1991) work as the most theoretically robust health promotion framework when tested against the criteria in Boxes 2.1 and 2.2 and the competing frameworks in Chapters 2, 3 and 4. The next step in developing a nursing health promotion framework was to test the degree of fit between the nurse as behaviour change agent, the nurse as empowerment facilitator and the nurse as strategic practitioner (Piper 2004, 2007a) and the health promotion models in the Beattie (1991), and by implication the Piper and Brown (1998a) and Piper (2000), frameworks. Piper (2004) revealed that, although the fit was not absolute in all cases, a conceptual relationship was apparent including congruence between the socio-political and socio-cultural foundations and the Beattie (1993) models of health and cultural bias. This adds depth, strength and clarity to the analysis on the degree of fit and assists in conceptualising, contextualising and synthesising a health promotion framework for nursing.

Thus, the framework of health promotion nursing (Figure 5.1) is a form of derived (as opposed to borrowed or developed) theory. Historically, the process and means of developing theory in nursing has been characterised by long-standing debate on the merits of developing theory for understanding, explaining and prescribing nursing practice or on borrowing and applying theory from other disciplines (Meleis 2007). More latterly, the concept and practice of theory derivation, a mid-point on the theory development continuum, has emerged.

The ultimate goal for proponents of practice theory development is situation-producing theory (as explained in Chapter 2). This is the construction of action-oriented usable theory that, in shaping rather than just observing reality, can be applied to the practice setting and produce desirable patient or nursing practice outcomes (Meleis 2007). It both emanates from and guides nursing practice.

Borrowed theory is where theory is developed by another discipline and used in its original and unmodified form in nursing (Walker and Avant 2005). Johnson (1968) sees the differentiation between borrowed and unique theory (the process and outcome of theory development unique to a discipline) as unhelpful. She takes the view that, as neither can endure and any division between the sciences is arbitrary, knowledge defies artificial boundaries and is not owned by any one discipline. Cormack and Reynolds (1992) concur in seeing nursing as an applied science and thus theory can be borrowed from other disciplines if it assists nursing practice.

Conversely, Johnson (1968), Walker (1971) and Phillips (1977) contend that if nursing research is undertaken from the perspective of borrowed theory from other subject areas, this may serve the cause of science and of these disciplines but not necessarily the cause or scientific development of nursing. It could also give the impression that nursing has no specific knowledge-base of its own (Parse 1999).

The problem, as Donaldson and Crowley (1978) see it, is that theory generated by a discipline reflects the unique context and criteria for knowledge within that field and may mean it is not readily transferable for use elsewhere. In addition, the process of borrowing theory from other disciplines and not reconceptualising it to fit the nursing perspective may obstruct questions being asked that are of specific concern to nursing. This slows up the development of unique nursing science and inhibits the generation of theory from a nursing frame of reference (Phillips 1977). Nevertheless, for many this dependence on other disciplines for knowledge and the use of borrowed theory remains a key feature of nursing (Mitchell 1992).

Unique theory development in nursing can only come about through asking research questions and studying phenomena in a way that is not characteristic of any other discipline (Johnson 1968). This is difficult for nursing as its research foundations and circumscribed body of knowledge are still developing (Johnson 1974; Parse 1999). In addition, if disciplines are characterised by a unique perspective and world view that define the boundaries of their research (Donaldson and Crowley 1978), the use of borrowed theory is similarly problematic.

Borrowed theory and theory derivation share a resemblance in using the theory from another discipline as their starting point. However, theory derivation differs in taking, in this case, a factor-relating theory (as per Chapter 2), i.e. a health promotion framework (Health Promotion Theory 1) from its original field of inquiry (Field 1) and, as the two fields are different, modifies, synthesises, redefines and restates concepts as required so that it fits with, and is meaningful to nursing (Field 2). This forms a new theory (Theory 2) which offers insight into the new discipline (Walker and Avant 2005), i.e. nursing. This process, based on a modified version of Walker and Avant's (2005) diagram, is illustrated in Figure 5.2.

Thus, theory for use in theory derivation is selected from another discipline on the basis of its potential usefulness in explaining, describing or predicting particular phenomena of interest for nursing. Its purpose and value is in enabling new insight to be gained and explanation to be given about phenomena that are poorly understood, insufficiently robust in terms of theory development or where there is a dearth of literature and formal study (Walker and Avant 2005).

Using existing theory in this way allows nursing to take advantage of advances in other fields of inquiry while addressing their research to another problem (Cleland 1967). It becomes nursing theory when the process of derivation and synthesis reconceptualises existing theory and gives new meaning to nursing phenomena and nursing problems from a nursing perspective (Meleis 2007) or nursing frame of reference (Phillips 1977). It becomes nursing research when the inquiry is undertaken from a nursing perspective (Donaldson and Crowley 1978). It is not who developed the theory or where it was developed that matters, the crux is that it is being used to address nursing phenomena (Meleis 2007).

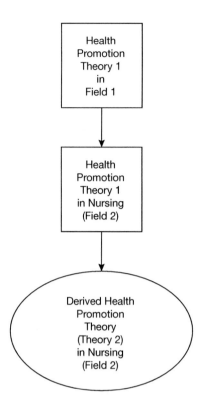

Figure 5.2 The process of theory derivation (after Walker and Avant 2005)

The health promotion framework of this book (Figure 5.1) derives, then, from intersecting unique, generated theory from Piper's (2004) research findings with borrowed theory, i.e. Beattie's 1991 health promotion framework (informed by Beattie 1993; Douglas 1982; Piper and Brown 1998a; Piper 2000, 2004, 2007a, 2007b). It represents a process of making sense of phenomena in nursing through analogy from another discipline (Walker and Avant 2005). Testing the themes and findings of Piper's (2004) research and the nursing health promotion framework in Figure 5.1 against Walker and Avant's (2005) list of iterative procedures (Box 5.2) helps illustrate further how theory derivation has been achieved and the nursing health promotion framework developed. Although the way in which the procedures are presented suggests a sequential process, the authors point out that the process is more likely to be iterative. In other words, there is movement backwards and forwards between the procedures until the desired level of sophistication is attained.

BOX 5.2 THEORY DERIVATION PROCEDURES

- Thorough familiarity with the pertinent literature and the level of theory development in nursing and an evaluation of the relative merits of this work as demonstrated in Chapter 4. As none of this latter theory was fit for purpose then theory derivation was able to proceed.
- Thorough familiarity with the pertinent literature and the means of theory development in relation to the topic under scrutiny in both nursing and other disciplines, as demonstrated in Chapters 2 and 3.
- The selection of a parent theory (Beattie's 1991 health promotion framework) for theory derivation and an outline of its Theory 1 in Field 1 format as in Chapter 2. The criteria for the selection of the parent theory included its ability to offer new insight into, and a structure for conceptualising and contextualising nursing health promotion. The latter was assisted by Beattie (1993), Douglas (1982), Piper and Brown (1998a) and Piper (2000, 2004, 2007a, 2007b).
- The content and structure of the parent theory that was used and that best fits nursing were clearly identified (see Chapters 2, 5, 6, 7, 8 and 9).
- The concepts and structure of the parent theory were modified, redefined and restated so that they are meaningful to, and fit with the new field of inquiry. Phillips (1977) emphasises that the theory cannot be simply transposed without being reconceptualised and synthesised from a nursing frame of reference, as in the nursing health promotion framework in Figure 5.1.

(Walker and Avant 2005)

CONCLUSION

This chapter has outlined how the themes and deviant/paradigm cases of inductive, qualitative research findings and use of theory from another subject area have generated a derived health promotion framework for nursing (Figure 5.1). This is important because although the health and professional policy and nursing literature identifies health promotion as an important element of practice, the development of a specific, multipurpose framework that can be used to identify, plan and contextualise clinically focused interventions, strategic and patient-led processes and any related consensus are notably absent. The knowledge, power base and aims, processes, impact, outcomes and evaluatory criteria of the nurse as behaviour change agent, the nurse as empowerment facilitator and the nurse as strategic practitioner enumerated by the framework in relation to individual and macro/ micro patient population foci of intervention have also been articulated. These are further developed in Chapters 6, 7, 8 and 9 in Part 2 of the book, which focuses on practice.

LEARNING TRIGGERS

Having read Chapter 5, complete the learning triggers below to reinforce your understanding of the concepts that have been discussed:

- Summarise the key features of the health promotion framework advanced in Figure 5.1.
- Identify the relationship between the health promotion models within Figure 5.1.
- Describe briefly how the above were developed from qualitative research themes and theory derivation.
- Describe briefly the sequential process of theory derivation.
- List examples of health promotion models evaluation indicators from the input, process, impact and outcome categories.

PART 2

PRACTICE

THE NURSE AS BEHAVIOUR CHANGE AGENT

6

INTRODUCTION

This chapter focuses on the indicators and practical (i.e. not just the ideological/theoretical) examples of the nurse as behaviour change agent in the form of the aims, processes, impact, outcomes and evaluation criteria of intervention of this traditional model of nurse-led health promotion. Primary, secondary and tertiary health promotion are discussed together with the nature of behaviour change, communication and behaviour change theory, compliance, adherence, concordance and the 'medical model' and its associated socio-political values.

LEARNING OUTCOMES

By reading this chapter, and completing the learning triggers at the end, the reader should have a better understanding of:

- the nurse as behaviour change agent model of health promotion;
- the aims, processes, impact and evaluation criteria and outcomes of intervention;
- compliance, adherence and concordance;
- primary health promotion and targeted outreach;
- secondary and tertiary health promotion;
- communication and behaviour change theory;
- the medical model, its associated socio-political values and its relationship to the nurse as behaviour change agent.

In essence, the nurse as behaviour change agent aims to achieve predetermined behavioural outcomes based on the assessment of health risks and/or needs and problems by the nurse. It is a core element of health care activity (Whitehead and Russell 2004) and is based on the assumption that health-related behaviour is a key determinant of health/disease (Crossley 2001). It also assumes that individuals are free to choose their health/disease-related behaviour and lifestyle. Findings from Piper (2004) indicate that success is measured by the degree of compliance and self-management and is achieved through top-down awareness-raising and patient teaching. It includes educating people on the correct use of services, i.e. right patient, right place, right time and keeping those that the nurse deems appropriate in the system. It was also suggested in Piper's (2004) study that reassuring patients about the quality and genuineness of health care professionals to help achieve patient co-operation and make it easier for doctors to do their job was part of the role.

The premise of the nurse as behaviour change agent is that the health of people will be improved by their understanding the relationship between physical and mental disease, risk factors and lifestyle. The UK Prime Minister's Strategy Unit/Cabinet Office (Halpern *et al.* 2004) contends that health outcomes are strongly related to lifestyle choices, for example diet, exercise, smoking and alcohol consumption.

As was seen in Figure 5.1, in this scenario the power and thus the locus of control of the nurse is high and this is reinforced by technical expertise and objective, scientific and medical knowledge. Thus, the nurse as behaviour change agent prescribes behaviour and aspects of lifestyle in the context of specific disease or perceived health risks while adopting a 'high social distance' (Beattie 1991: 185). The emphasis is on the need to get individuals to control and regulate their health-related behaviour and correct any inadequacies and deficits by highlighting the health risks they face if they fail to pursue the prescribed course of action. It is assumed that individuals are free to make rational, conscious decisions about their health-related behaviour and lifestyle and that these are the primary determinant of disease. For Piper and Brown (1998b), Beattie (1991) refers to this type of health promotion as health persuasion techniques advisedly, as it represents an attempt to impose and socially reinforce external beliefs.

PRIMARY HEALTH PROMOTION

Primary, i.e preventive, health promotion aims to prevent disease and injury and promote biological homeostasis and body self-regulation by disseminating health information selectively derived from medically related research to individuals about risk factors and associated behaviour. This involves nurses in supporting the one-way messages of large scale, high profile, mass media awareness-raising campaigns on health topics or the correct use of health services. The public are confronted with all manner of images including those designed to scare and of what might happen if they fail to conform and adopt a healthy lifestyle (Seedhouse 1997). Health is presented as a state of risk (Gastaldo 1997) with everything a potential source of that risk and with everyone at risk (Peterson 1997). The aim is to trigger 'do-it-yourself' attitude and then behaviour/lifestyle changes consistent with the recommended advice given.

For Whitehead (2000), mass communication/media campaigns are a powerful way to disseminate persuasive health promotion messages to target groups, including those that are hard to reach, but nursing has been slow to adopt this approach. He acknowledges that the lack of personal feedback makes it difficult to 'tailor' the message to the specific needs of individual patients and clients, that such intervention is impersonal and that nurses, who are used to face-to-face health promotion, may feel that it is unsuitable practice for nursing. Nevertheless, he feels that the potential benefits outweigh the disadvantages. He urges nurses to become more active users of this type of primary health promotion, while later acknowledging the potential for underestimating the scale and the complexity of this facet of practice within the confines of the nursing role (Whitehead and Russell 2004). Whitehead (2000) outlines the means by which mass media campaigns are most likely to be effective (Box 6.1).

As an example, Piper (2007b) outlines how this works from an emergency-nurse perspective. It includes themed displays, leaflets in display racks, posters and health promotion videos showing in the emergency department waiting room and strategically placed elsewhere in the department on a variety of topics aimed at patients and those that accompany them. These might be on accident prevention, first aid, the dangers of alcohol misuse, smoking, risk factors for coronary heart disease (CHD) or cancer or on healthy eating that tie in with national and international initiatives such as Drinkwise Day or World Aids Day. Similarly, Whitehead *et al.* (2004) report campaigning to prevent osteoporosis via displays for the general public in the main concourse of the hospital and in high-profile areas in clinical settings.

However, although effective at raising awareness about health risks, it is important to acknowledge that if operating as a sole strategy for health-related behaviour change the outcomes are likely to be at best uncertain (Naidoo and Wills 2000; Whitehead and Russell 2004). If the campaign is too generalised and engages in stereotyping it is also likely to be ignored by the population to whom it is directed (McEwan and Bhopal 1991).

The UK Prime Minister's Strategy Unit/Cabinet Office accept that copious research over the years has shown that the provision of information and guidance, i.e. knowledge alone via 'weak' mediums such as leaflets, often fails to change the health-related behaviour of much of the population (Halpern *et al.* 2004). They advance that it might be wiser to focus more on stronger agents of persuasion such as nurses to influence health-related behaviour due to the high esteem in which they are held and their involvement at life-defining moments.

Whitehead and Russell (2004) note that it is important not to under-estimate the complexity of changing an individual's lifestyle, that to do so requires concerted, methodical intervention for any measure of success. They add that some people simply do not want to change and defer responding to the implications of unhealthy behaviour. The Strategy Unit/Cabinet Office share this view and refer to:

- the psychology of discounting – where immediate gratification takes precedence over potential long-term gain;
- the attraction of high and varying impact experiences over those that are more constant;
- and losses having a greater impact than comparable gains.

(Halpern et al. 2004)

In addition, health-related behaviour change often requires the giving up of something that is pleasurable and habitual and can be an uncomfortable process, and individuals may use information selectively to justify their current behaviour by shutting out anything that conflicts with their lifestyle. This may be compounded by the nurse imposing health messages on people, which would both undermine individual autonomy and be ethically questionable. Thus, simply to expect individuals to change their behaviour in response to objective information about the possibility of disease without taking account of social variables etc is naive (Whitehead 2001b).

As the UK Strategy Unit/Cabinet Office observes:

> several powerful psychological forces are ranged against public health professionals. Discounting makes us disinclined to change our behaviour now for a long-term gain in health or longevity (rather the burger today than the extra year tomorrow). Asymmetry of losses versus gains make us disinclined to give up our current satisfaction (smoking) for a potential gain (feeling fitter). And our psychological defences and attributions make us feel that early death and morbidity are things that happen to others, not us.

(Halpern et al. 2004: 39).

They contend that health care professionals need to understand these factors both to help change individual health-related behaviour and also to galvanise public support for primary health promotion programmes. They also highlight how attitudes to health-related behaviour change over time. They contrast the public support for the compulsory wearing of seatbelts today with the initial public resistance to this legislation in the 1970s; how in the past it would have been unthinkable to ban smoking on aircraft whereas now it would be inconceivable to allow it; and a softening of attitudes toward prostitution.

Primary health promotion also includes targeted outreach such as the contraceptive service for young people described by Baraitser *et al.* (2002). The idea is to reach out to vulnerable or target groups who are deemed by health professionals to be at risk and find ways to facilitate their use of a particular health service. A similar example would be drug outreach work targeting difficult to reach drug users with harm-minimisation interventions (clean needles, syringes, sterile water, etc.) with the ultimate intention of finding strategies to get them to come in to the clinic and ultimately on to detoxification programmes.

Baraitser *et al.* (2002) set out to establish a relationship between the clinic and local organisations working with young people (including schools) on issues of school truancy, youth offending, adventurer play and work experience for those under-performing at school. They identify what they consider to be 'innovative' ways of working to help maximise the likelihood of young people accessing their service. These include:

- linking clinics to a local community;
- being proactive, i.e. creating and updating a database of local organisations, regularly contacting these and offering a flexible health promotion programme;
- specifically employing a family planning nurse as outreach worker (in preference to any other) so that even at the first point of contact people are meeting a clinician with expert sexual health knowledge and a thorough knowledge of how local services operate.

They claimed that they increased the use of family planning services overall, but particularly among their target group, through a combination of targeted outreach, extended clinic hours and open access/drop-in services and that this suggests a previously unmet need for quality contraceptive services. As a result of working closely with schools, having knowledge and skills needed to access the clinic as learning objectives in sex education classes and having some lessons clinic-based providing an opportunity for pupils to meet clinic staff, young people were made well aware of the services, how they work and what they offer.

Goold *et al.* (2006) found that young people were quite well informed about sexually transmitted infections but not about what services were available to treat them. They recommend greater involvement by the client group to help find ways to address this anomaly. However, it is important to be mindful of any potential difference of perspective when developing services. For example, Chambers *et al.* (2002) found something of a discrepancy between what young people considered important and the views of health care professionals for reducing teenage pregnancy. The former were concerned with young person-centred interventions and suggested more creative ways of disseminating sexual health promotion messages than did health care professionals, with the latter medicalising the issue and emphasising the importance of service-based solutions, i.e. the organisation of dedicated young people's sexual health and education services.

In addition, Whitehead (2005c) warns about counter attitudinal behaviour by young people in defiance of top-down health promotion campaigns on emotionally charged topics such as illicit drug use or sexual activity that endeavour to deny an important part of a young person's health experience. In Whitehead's view (2005c), many young people are well informed about what can jeopardise their health and make informed and rational judgements about risk. After cost-benefit analysis they may still opt to engage in behaviour that may put their short- or long-term health at risk as part of a process of experimentation and expression of individual identity. For some, this may have serious consequences but health promotion campaigns may have no impact on these individuals. Indeed, negative and risk-focused campaigning may also make high-risk behaviour seem more exciting and serve to entice rather than dissuade participation. Unsafe sex, excessive drinking, smoking and drug use have a certain cachet precisely because of their association with risk-taking and rejection of accepted cultural mores (Crossley 2001).

Thus, Whitehead (2005c) contends that intervention must take account of and dovetail with the attitude and belief systems of young people and wonders if it might not be better for health promotion intervention to try to make the experience as safe as possible (harm minimisation). The role of empowerment, peer education and health-promoting school strategies are acknowledged and the creation of supportive, safe environments within which young people flirt with attenuated risk is advocated. This is because attempts to prevent risk-taking are notoriously ineffective and might be perceived as the efforts of killjoys (Whitehead 2005c).

Nelson and Ruth (1998) used a similar targeted outreach approach to that of Baraitser *et al.* (2002) and what they called 'proactive' health promotion. They worked with local primary schools to raise accident awareness in children and to provide insight into the workings of an accident and emergency department. They aimed to help demystify the service, reduce anxiety if the children needed treatment in the future and build further links with the community. They used role-play, practical sessions with plaster of paris, bandages, blood pressure machines and X-ray equipment and a work sheet for completion at home with parents.

SECONDARY AND TERTIARY HEALTH PROMOTION

Piper (2007b) uses emergency nursing and the emergency department to help illustrate secondary and tertiary health promotion. Secondary health promotion is concerned with patients discharged home from the emergency department and with compliance with prescribed treatment regimes specifically related to their presenting problem. The goal of patient self-management of injury and disease is to maximise chances of full recovery, restoration of function and to minimise the risk of complications or relapse. The emergency nurse determines the specific behaviour(s) required and supplies the appropriate information, discharge advice, reassurance and patient teaching to achieve this. For example, information and advice on how to care for a fractured limb in a plaster cast, a sprained ankle or minor head injury, the potential complications and what rehabilitative behaviours the patient can adopt. This is reinforeced by an information sheet that the patient and their significant others can take away for reference, and the emergency department contact telephone number should a problem arise.

Tertiary health promotion operates along the same lines as secondary but when working with patients presenting with exacerbations of chronic problems. The issues for consideration are likely to be more complex, and more-detailed health promotion input may be provided by health care professionals from without the department such as clinical nurse specialists/nurse consultants prior to discharge. It may also be that the severity of the exacerbation demands emergency admission and thus health promotion of the type described above may be problematic, ineffective and inappropriate.

More generally, the UK Department of Health (2006a) is keen to introduce social prescribing, i.e. information prescriptions for those with enduring (chronic) illness. They give exercise-on-prescription schemes as an example and refer to 'well-being' prescriptions to promote good health and independence and greater access to a range of services and activities.

For Piper and Brown (1998a), secondary and tertiary health promotion includes the provision of disease-specific and discharge information as well as information about community services to patients. Betz (2006) refers to evidence of effective surgical preoperative preparation of children to help reduce stress and thus maximise surgical outcome, advancing that intervention needs to incorporate age-specific information on what can be expected from the surgical experience. Other factors to consider are the timing of the intervention, previous surgical experiences of the child and the severity of their condition.

Robinson and Miller (1996) highlight that the stress and pressure of being in hospital and being ill compromise effective communication. In response to this and large numbers of telephone enquiries from parents of children discharged home from an orthopaedic ward, they explored the content and language of written information relating to care of a plaster cast at home. They subsequently developed a jargon free, 'plain English' set of discharge instructions.

The problem with the primary, secondary and tertiary health promotion interventions of the nurse as behaviour change agent, which are orientated towards the individual and involve health-related learning, is that the process can model a top-down and didactic rather than a listening nurse–patient relationship (Macleod Clark *et al.* 1991). The emphasis on professionally determined needs may not only overlook the patient's perception of needs or achieve their participation in care but also reinforces the power base of the nurse and engenders patient deference and dependence.

The nurse as behaviour change agent then, as Piper and Brown (1998a) point out, invokes a range of health promotion interventions that involve the dissemination of information to either the general public or patients/clients or, for school nurses, pupils in a variety of social contexts (hospitals, schools, health centres, etc.). The focus is on primary prevention, health service use or how best to manage an existing disease, injury or disability, whether in acute or chronic form, for maximum rehabilitation and prevention of deterioration, complications or relapse. The aims, methods and evaluation criteria in the form of impact (intermediate outcome) and outcome of the nurse as behaviour change agent are summarised in Table 6.1.

COMMUNICATION AND BEHAVIOUR CHANGE THEORY

As Piper (2007) points out, health promotion of this ilk can be thought of as a simple communication process, which has been likened to an

Table 6.1 The nurse as behaviour change agent

Aims	Process	Impact evaluation indicators	Outcome evaluation indicators
Primary prevention	Mass-media campaigns e.g. smoking, cycle helmets, exercise, etc.	Change in health-related behaviour, i.e. reduction in 'risk factors'	Reduction in: mortality morbidity complications relapse
Secondary and tertiary prevention	Targeted outreach	Compliance with treatment regimes	
Appropriate use of services	Verbal and written instructions on: injury/disease management complications, etc.	Self-management by patient in use of needle exchange schemes	
	Pre and post treatment expectations		
	Patient teaching e.g. injection technique for newly diagnosed diabetics	Uptake of services	
		Right patient, right place, right time	
	Supplementary discharge advice		
	Needle exchange schemes		
	Patient information about services		

electrical system model by Hills (1979). Although this undermines the complexity of the nurse–patient interpersonal interaction by reducing it to a mechanistic relationship, it serves a purpose and can be illustrated as follows:

Input > Coding > Channel > Decoding > Output

The nurse provides the input and the coding and the patient/client is the decoder. The method is concerned with the sender validating and transmitting health promotion information to the receiver (patient) with the latter feeding back on how the sender's messages have been received, decoded and understood and the course of action the patient/client is proposing to take (output). Ewles and Shipster (1984) summarise this as a three-stage process involving giving information or advice to a patient/client about their injury/disease and ensuring that they understand it, remember it and can act on it. They stress the need to define the objectives and intended outcomes for the intervention, to give the information in a structured way emphasising and repeating the important aspects, and the need to use short words and short sentences to avoid any misunderstanding. Whitehead and Russell (2004) add that it is important for nurses to avoid overloading patients with information, to assess previous health behaviours and not to set unrealistic goals.

However, as Piper and Brown (1998b), Whitehead (2001b) and Crossley (2001) point out, primary health promotion campaigns aimed at achieving health-related learning (Tones and Tilford 2001) and attitude and lifestyle change are underpinned by more sophisticated theories and models of health-related behaviour drawn from psychology. These seek to understand, describe and explain what knowledge, perceptions, beliefs, values and social norms motivate an individual's health-related behaviour and any actions taken to avoid disease in relation to perceived threat. They have been applied to problem eating, drinking, smoking, drug-use and sex in an attempt to predict health-related behaviour (Crossley 2001) and include social cognitive models (Whitehead 2001b), the Health Belief Model (Rosenstock et al. 1988) and the Theory of Reasoned Action (Fishbein and Ajzen 1985).

The Health Belief Model and the Theory of Reasoned Action reflect an acknowledgement of the limitations of simple communication models. They undermine the fallacy that the provision of health-related knowledge (K) alone will induce a change of attitude (A) and modification of behaviour (B) (KAB model) identified as necessary by the nurse as behaviour change agent. Whitehead and Russell (2004) fear that some nurses may base their practice on these very assumptions, hold the view that health-related behaviour change in individuals is easily achieved and highlight the need for nurses to be better informed about the limitations of this approach. In support of this position, Piper and Brown (1998b) cite Nutbeam and Blakey (1990) who contend that psychological models and theories are based on the premise that information provision alone has minimal effect on knowledge and behaviour. Even an enhanced knowledge base is unlikely to catalyse behaviour change if concomitant attitudes and beliefs are not modified. Successful behaviour-change interventions depend, at the very least, on a sound understanding of the complexities involved and the processes required (Whitehead 2001b).

The HBM posits that health-related behaviours are the product of perceived susceptibility to health threats, the severity of the threats and costs and barriers to change. They are based on the rationalistic premise that health-related behaviour stems from an assessment of the potential costs and benefits of behaviour together with the influence of subjective norms such as parental and peer pressure (Crossley 2001). The Theory of Reasoned Action/Planned Behaviour (TPB) contends that the best way to predict behaviour is by measuring intention (i.e. attitude), subjective norm and perceived control over behaviour. Attitude is defined as an individual's positive or negative evaluation of behaviour, which is judged to be indicative of beliefs held about the outcome of the behaviour (Giles *et al.* 2005).

Giles *et al.* (2005) provide an example of how the TPB was used to predict and explain condom use in African adolescents and the role played by individual and group factors in a rural location. They claim strong support for the predictive power of the TPB but found no evidence to directly link attitudes towards condoms to their use. They highlight the strength of family/social influences on sexual behaviour and related decision-making. Thus, they question health promotion activities that focus solely on individual behaviour change and stress the need for interventions to also penetrate community networks.

Piper and Brown (1998a) cite Galvin's (1992) use of the Theory of Reasoned Action at a secondary level to achieve smoking cessation among patients. Thus, they (Piper and Brown 1998a) acknowledge that primary/secondary health promotion is an important part of nursing practice and that psychology legitimately provides a theoretical base underpinning intervention. Their concern is that these ostensibly 'neutral' models and theories are deployed without consideration of their ideological/philosophical standpoint and what this means for nurse–patient power relations.

Intervention attempts to impose and reinforce external beliefs and to use various cues, for example mass media campaigns, to trigger KAB. It is simplistic, information-based intervention underpinned by health psychology for behaviour change. Health and risk are often portrayed as black or white and health promotion messages as scientifically objective interventions encouraging value-free choices to, what is believed to be, a largely passive public waiting to be directed on how best to lead a safe, healthy life in accordance with these edicts (Crossley 2001). The problem for health promoters, and thus nurses, is that health-related behavioural choices are seldom this clear cut and are clouded by uncertainties and ambiguities but, even if it was this straightforward, the public are certainly not (Crossley 2001).

Piper and Brown (1998a) see this as medicalised and rationalistic health promotion and a philosophy of psychological determinism which fails to acknowledge the impact of social context on human action. Crossley (2001) concurs in contending that in focusing solely on cognitive processes and individual behaviour change, the theories and models of psychology have failed to provide a sophisticated understanding of underlying meanings and how these relate to morality and the socio-economic context of health-related behaviour. The recognition that disease is caused by a complex mixture of biological, psychological and social causes is a direct challenge to the medical model of health (Crossley 2001).

COMPLIANCE, ADHERENCE AND CONCORDANCE

The concept of compliance fits with the top-down, expert-directed and an almost coercive nurse as behaviour change agent. Compliance means patients doing as they are told by the nurse and obeying instructions in relation to treatment regimes (Hobden 2006a) at a secondary/tertiary level, and lifestyle issues (Vermeire et al. 2001) from a primary health promotion perspective, as discussed above. As such, compliance has come to be linked with submissive behaviour and Piper (2004) notes that participants in his study talked about getting patients to change their views, take tablets correctly and do things the way nurses thought they should.

It is almost like accepting punishment and has thus developed negative connotations with non-compliance seen by some as an enduring and complex problem. Indeed poor compliance is expected in 30–50 per cent of patients, particularly in those with chronic disease (Vermeire et al. 2001) such as diabetes (Hall 2006). Non-compliance may be intentional, i.e. a deliberate decision not to follow instructions and take medication as prescribed, or unintentional (Hobden 2006a). In failing or refusing to comply, and thus exhibiting irrational behaviour from the perspective of the health care professional, it is assumed the patient is relinquishing the opportunity to receive therapy that will be good for them (Vermeire *et al.* 2001). With reference to the literature, Vermeire *et al.* (2001) identify the categories of non-compliance outlined in Box 6.2 but find it more difficult to state precisely the causes. None of the more obvious indicators from the literature, namely:

- type of disease
- clinical setting
- type of treatment
- age
- sex
- marital status
- social class

are definitive indicators of non-compliance.

Potential indicators include mental health problems, memory loss, duration and complexity of treatment and associated side effects, the number, cost and frequency of medications, being asymptomatic and any of the patient's unresolved anxieties. Sherman (2007) concurs with side effects and adds that patient perceptions of taking too many and/or unnecessary medications are additional factors to consider. Equally, if not more important is the quality of communication between the health care professional and the patient and the quality

BOX 6.2 CATEGORIES OF NON-COMPLIANCE

- delay in seeking care;
- not participating in health programmes;
- failure to keep appointments;
- not having a prescription made up (primary non-compliance);
- not taking the correct dose of medication;
- taking medication at the wrong time;
- forgetting to take medication;
- stopping treatment too soon;
- failing to get a repeat prescription (secondary non-compliance).

(Vermeire *et al.* 2001)

of their interpersonal relationship (Donovan and Blake 1992; Vermeire *et al.* 2001; Campbell *et al.* 2007) and its effect on patient satisfaction (Campbell *et al.* 2007). It is also important to remember that patients do a cost-benefit analysis, i.e. they weigh up the pros and cons of taking medication based on their knowledge, attitudes, experience and social context (Donovan and Blake 1992; Vermeire *et al.* 2001; Hobden 2006a). Compliance may be enhanced by the use of better labelling, calendars, special containers that have pre-assembled drug combinations for specific times of the day, written and oral information (Vermeire *et al.* 2001).

Conversely, adherence represents negotiated outcomes, i.e. co-operation and partnership (Vermeire *et al.* 2001). With adherence patients keep to a treatment agreement established between them and the health care professional with non-adherence meaning that they renege on the agreement (Hobden 2006a). Concordance is driven by patient led/defined outcomes. Adherence and concordance are more consistent with empowering practice, patient satisfaction and the nature of the consultation (Hobden 2006a) as per Chapter 7.

Social context

As has been seen, the nurse as behaviour change agent emphasises the need for individuals to control health risks. It assumes that individuals are free to choose their health-related behaviour and that lifestyle is the primary cause of ill-health, i.e. that health-related decision-making is a value-free intellectual act independent of emotional and social influences (Rush 1997). This overlooks the fact that health, as a social product, is influenced by socio-economic inequalities (Townsend *et al.* 1992; Acheson 1998) and is compatible with a health and social policy stance of minimal state intervention (Beattie (1993).

Piper and Brown (1998a) cite Rodmell and Watt's (1986) assertion that health-related behaviour decisions are influenced by physical surroundings over which individuals may have little control. They also refer to Mitchell (1982) who highlights the challenge of, for example, giving up smoking if financial circumstances dictate this to be an individual's only luxury, or the futility of giving up smoking to live longer when there is no prospect of a job. They conclude that a combination of structural (physical and economic) and cultural (value systems) factors that undermine the opportunity to exercise healthy lifestyle choices means that it may well be unrealistic to expect individuals to change their behaviour from what might be appropriate to their environment to that advocated by nurses. From a socio-cultural perspective, Beattie (1993) links efforts to force behaviour change with a culture of subordination concerned with order and social regulation, conformity and compliance and thus the medical model.

THE NURSE AS BEHAVIOUR CHANGE AGENT AND THE MEDICAL MODEL

The inception of the medical model can be traced back to the Cartesian revolution and the development of germ theory. For Descartes the mind and the body were separate independent entities. He viewed the body purely as physical substance subordinate in nature to the mind. While the mind, as the seat of the soul, remained the province of religion, the emphasis on the physical nature of the body enabled it to be seen simply in mechanistic and reductionist terms (Hart 1985). The isolated, individual body became a legitimate focus for detached, objective positivistic science and medicine leading to the development of germ theory linking the aetiology of disease to micro-organisms (Vuori 1980; Hart 1985). It is both mechanistic and reductionist and reflects an ideological position, i.e. a set of values and beliefs.

The traditional critique of the ideological stance of the medical model characterises it as an institution of social control (Zola 1972; Crawford 1977, 1980; Hart 1985; Ballard and Elston 2005). The argument put forward is that while claiming to be a value-free science medicine reinforces the social class structure and social order via the asymmetrical health care professional–patient inter-personal relationship and primary health promotion campaigns that act as a form of propaganda encouraging compliance with prescribed therapy. Social problems are translated into individual, disease-related, decontextualised problems and medical solutions are advanced (Vuori 1980; Caraher 1994c, 1995; Lowenberg 1995; Ballard and Elston 2005).

This rationalistic premise holds that reason and health-related decision-making are also value-free intellectual acts independent of emotional and social influences (Rush 1997). Occupational stress due to work pressures, for example, then becomes a lifestyle problem and the fault of the worker (Crawford 1977; Lowenberg 1995; Rush 1997). This ideology of individual responsibility not only obscures the class structure of work and the economic roots of illness (Crawford 1977; Mitchell 1982), it absolves society for failing to meet the basic needs of some its people (Lowenberg 1995) and is 'victim-blaming' (Crawford 1977; Rush 1997). Tones and Green (2004) summarise the key aspects of the traditional medical model in Box 6.3.

Health is measured in terms of epidemiological and individual indicators, such as patterns of mortality and morbidity, and the absence of the signs and symptoms of disease. This model emphasises cause and effect at the individual level (Brown and Piper 1997). Health promotion intervention endeavours to find individual solutions to actual or potential medicalised problems by translating them into signs and symptoms and individual dysfunction amenable to preventive intervention and/or treatment. It is disease- rather than person-centred (Seedhouse 1997).

Medical model/primary health promotion emphasises risk aversion in individuals, encourages self-discipline and body management through the personal regulation of health-related behaviour (Crawford 1977; Lupton 1997) with or without therapeutic help. Crossley (2001) advances that the concept of health here has taken on moral as well as ideological connotations. Indeed the Strategy Unit/Cabinet Office (Halpern *et al.* 2004) contend that there are strong moral and political arguments for accepting personal responsibility for health and related behaviour, that enhancing personal responsibility is an inherently good thing and about moral fibre and character. The problem for Crossley (2001) is that this translates into value judgements about good and correct behaviour and she asks where this leaves those engaging in apparent high-risk behaviour such as smoking, eating 'junk' food, or having unsafe sex? Do these simply reflect irrational individual choices or do they represent a complementary rationality and stand, for example, as symbols of trust, intimacy and love among gay men who have unsafe sex?

The medical model perspective is accepted by the social construc-tionist/Foucauldian perspective, but only as a partial representation of reality. Social constructionists concur in part that medicine is an objective, factual, detached science that reflects a social and political belief system that transforms social problems into disease. They also

---

BOX 6.3 A SUMMARY OF THE KEY ASPECTS OF THE MEDICAL MODEL

- viewing the body as a machine (mechanistic);
- separating the mind and the body (dualism);
- focusing on the biomedical cause of disease (pathogenesis);
- relating specific disease to specific causes (cause and effect).

(Tones and Green 2004)

believe that medicine does exercise disciplinary power and is an agent of social control, but that the medicalisation of everyday life (May 1992; Lupton 1997) is also done in a constructive rather than a repressive way (Ballard and Elston 2005).

The social constructionist/Foucauldian literature stresses that patient–health care professional power relations are not a symbol of class conflict with the latter striving to assert their power base to reinforce the established social order and their place in the hierarchy. Although links in a chain of power relations, health care professional dominance is based on collusion between the parties and willing complicity by patients and clients rather than coercion and repression by doctors and nurses, etc. The perpetuation of social inequalities through the nurse/doctor–patient consultation, with patients depicted as helpless, powerless victims unable to resist the might of the health care professions has been exaggerated. It overlooks the help and the benefits to health that health care professionals provide for their patients (Lupton 1997; Ballard and Elston 2005). Indeed, patients do not necessarily fulfil a passive, dependant role and use the medical model by lobbying for their experience of illness to be publicly validated by its representatives (Ballard and Elston 2005). The limitations of the power health care professionals have over patients' actions are also evidenced by poor compliance rates and disease management (Lupton 1997).

However, both the medical model and the Foucauldian concepts of medicalisation (Lupton 1997) and bio-power (Gastaldo 1997) contend that the clinical gaze of medicine has expanded to encompass both the sick and the potentially sick. This places everyone under medical surveillance to a greater or lesser extent and makes everyone a patient or potential patient. Health then becomes an 'at risk' state (Gastaldo 1997). As a result patients are required to divulge not only symptoms of their body but also the symptoms of their life (Zola 1972).

For Crossley (2001), it is important to remember that health-related decision-making is complex and is linked to issues of self, identity and morality and involves the concept of lay rationality where values other than health (as defined, for example, by nurses) take precedence. She adds that such values may constitute personal survival strategies and ways of adapting to social life and that this is compounded by the tension between deferring gratification in line with health promotion campaigns and the pressure of our contemporary identity of consumer and immediate gratification.

The nurse as behaviour change agent fits with this paternalistic, medical model concept of healthism (Crawford 1980) and lifestylism

(Rodmell and Watt 1986). This perpetuates the illusion that preventable health problems are caused almost exclusively by the unhealthy behaviour, lifestyle choices, personal habits and failings of irresponsible individuals who smoke, consume a poor diet, fail to take adequate exercise or manage stress effectively. These lifestyle choices, human foibles and thus health are assumed to be under the control of individuals. The latter are not only free to change at will but have a moral responsibility to exercise such choice and learn the appropriate life skills compatible with the risk management edicts of the medical establishment.

Disease, then, is partially attributed to affluence and over-indulgence, with individuals responsible for making themselves unwell because of their poor lifestyle choices. Seedhouse (1997) points out that this form of health promotion is concerned with how to improve the measurable and quantifiable aspects of physical life and summarises the relationship between the medical model, health and health promotion as follows:

- health = absence of disease, injury and disability;
- disease, injury and disability are both inherently bad and bad because they prevent normal functioning;
- disease, injury and disability are disruptive and costly in terms of lost life opportunity, working days and medical treatment;
- as bad health is experienced by individuals, health promotion should target individual behaviours;
- the prevention of disease, injury and disability should be done where it will be effective and where it will not destabilise or disrupt society.

The purpose of unilateral fragmented health promotion campaigns focusing on specific diseases, or on medically defined problems and associated aspects of health-related behaviour, is also to get people to use the appropriate health services without questioning their relevance or effectiveness if disease ensues (Vuori 1980). Allied to this is the implication that if medically defined problems are the focus for intervention, then health professionals are the most suitable health promoters and the best time to undertake the process is when people are in contact with health services (Vuori 1980).

For Jones (1994), it is important to acknowledge that nurses willingly collude with, and are happy to act as agents of the medical model and exert control over patients. Any critique of the above has to take account of the ideological and organisational alliance between nursing and medicine and the way that nursing has contributed to the support and extension of medical power. In addition, by decontextualising disease from social processes imbalances in power between professional and patient are perpetuated and this helps maintain the nurse–patient hierarchy (Beattie 1991).

CONCLUSION

This chapter has presented a brief theoretical analysis and discussion on the nature, aim, processes, intended health outcomes and tensions of the nurse as behaviour change agent. As Piper and Brown (1998a) contend, although a crucial part of effective nursing practice as a form of secondary prevention and tertiary health promotion, the questionable effectiveness of primary prevention at a population level should confine it to a supplementary role. In addition, the emphasis on protecting individual patients/clients from damaging health-related behaviours is based on an agenda determined, directed and validated by the nurse and nursing priorities. Assumptions are also made about an individual's freedom to choose health-related behaviour while overlooking socio-economic inequalities, the political and physical environment, health as a social experience and emphasising personal responsibility, all of which reflect a medical model authoritarian stance to further reinforce this contention. Thus, the nurse as behaviour change agent conflicts with the contemporary emphasis on patient empowerment.

LEARNING TRIGGERS

Having read Chapter 6, complete the learning triggers below to reinforce your understanding of the concepts that have been discussed:

- Summarise the key features of the nurse as behaviour change agent model of health promotion.
- List examples of the aims, processes, impact and evaluation criteria and outcomes of intervention.
- Define compliance and differentiate between compliance, adherence and concordance.
- Define primary, secondary and tertiary health promotion.
- Summarise the key features of communication and behaviour change theory.
- Identify the key features of the medical model and its socio-political values.

THE NURSE AS EMPOWERMENT FACILITATOR

7

INDIVIDUAL ACTION PERSPECTIVE

INTRODUCTION

This chapter is concerned with the concept of the nurse as empowerment facilitator. As with the nurse as behaviour change agent, an individual action perspective is maintained but the focus is on process as much as on outcome, i.e. not on top-down, traditional, professionally determined behaviour change. It is about the nature of the relationship between the nurse and the patient/client, a more bottom-up, negotiated way of working and a shift in the locus of control from the former to the latter, as illustrated in the health promotion framework in Chapter 5. It pursues patient participation, a nurse–patient partnership or patient/client led, non-hierarchical, non-coercive practice and includes informed choice, adherence and concordance, shared decision-making and advocacy. The emphasis is on patient/client-centred active participation and thus the associated indicators of the health promotion aims, process, impact and evaluation criteria and outcomes of pragmatic empowerment, i.e. empowerment as a technology (Tones 2001). It represents a radical departure from traditional nurse–patient interaction (Devine 1993) and a humanistic ideology.

INDIVIDUAL EMPOWERMENT

Lewin and Piper (2007) highlight that empowerment has evolved from being an aspect of health improvement in the 1970s to a pervasive feature of the health and social care discourse in the 1990s (Skelton

1994; Gilbert 1995; Humphries 1996; Rodwell 1996) and is linked with contemporary clinical practice, teaching and research (Salmon and Hall 2004). It was a feature of feminist ideology (Gibson 1991; Chavasse 1992 Rodwell 1996; Kendall 1998), gay rights (Rodwell 1996), the radical civil rights and community action ideology of the 1960s and personal development movement of the 1970s (Kieffer 1984; Gibson 1991; Rissel 1994; Kendall 1998).

Empowerment thus became something of a fashionable buzzword (Chavasse 1992; Gomm 1993; Parsloe 1997), was seen as good and wholesome and associated with revered concepts such as freedom (Gomm 1993). Lovemore and Dann (2002) contend that it has become a catchall phrase and is applied to almost any facet of human activity and contexts, for example, girl power, people power, personal power, consumer power and patient empowerment. Further to this, it is linked with the concept of community, i.e. community empowerment, empowerment centre and empowerment zones (Lovemore and Dann 2002).

It became a stated aim of many health and social care organisations and of their research strategies (Gilbert 1995), has entered the language of health and social care management, professionals and service users alike (Gilbert 2001) and is now central to the developing consumer culture and moves to empower patients. Examples of developments in this direction in the UK include moves to promote actively an expert-patient persona in those with enduring (chronic) illness (DoH 2001), representation for patients via Patient Advice and Liaison Services (DoH 2002) and informed choice (DoH 2004a).

Lewin and Piper (2007) note that although various authors have endeavoured to define empowerment (Skelton 1994; Gilbert 1995; Jacob 1996; Rodwell 1996; Kuokkanen and Leino-Kilpi 2000; Byrt and Dooher 2002), its precise meaning remains elusive and contested. There is no agreed definition (Rappaport 1984; Gibson 1991; Rissel 1994; Parsloe 1997; Gilbert 2001) hence its operationalisation has been somewhat nebulous (Kettunen et al. 2001).

Thus, although there may be an implied consensus with Gomm's (1993) notion that empowerment suggests that some people have a surfeit of power and others a deficit, or are powerless (Rappaport 1984), and that the imbalance needs to be redressed, the term is used without conceptual clarification (Lovemore and Dann 2002). Empowerment then, masks deep conceptual differences (Gomm 1993; Rissel 1994; Parsloe 1997) and contradictions and its meaning depends on who is using it and the context in which it is being used (Rappaport 1984) and this adds to the ambiguity rather than clarity over its meaning (Lovemore and Dann 2002).

PATIENT INVOLVEMENT, PARTICIPATION, PARTNERSHIP AND SHARED DECISION-MAKING

Other important and related concepts that require consideration here are patient involvement/collaboration, patient participation, patient partnership and their hierarchical relationship (Cahill 1996) and shared decision-making (Charles et al. 2003). Patient involvement and patient collaboration fit with the more nurse-led, traditional nurse–patient relationship but are prerequisites for patient participation that is part of, but not synonymous with patient partnership. Both the latter are fundamental to nursing with patient partnership as the ideal that, for Cahill (1996), all nurses should be working towards.

The conclusion of UK Department of Health (2004c) research into patient and public involvement in health is that it delivers universally positive outcomes. They maintain that it increases patient satisfaction, confidence and trust, reduces anxiety and helps create better health care professional–patient relationships. It helps shape the policies, plans and services of the NHS and should be a central part of strategic planning and corporate responsibility.

Unlike the more sporadic patient participation, patient partnership demands closing the knowledge and information gap, complete and consistent patient involvement, a commitment to sharing all aspects of care and decision-making and an abdication of power by the nurse to achieve nurse–patient equality (Cahill 1996). In the main, patient partnership fits with shared decision-making as defined by Charles *et al.* (2003) in relation to early-stage breast cancer. They describe it as a process in which both the health care professional and the patient participate. Both are a complete departure from the traditional nurse as behaviour change agent type of approach where decisions are made for patients, information exchange is essentially one-way and there is almost no patient input other than informed consent (Charles *et al.* 2003).

Charles *et al.* (2003) differentiates between the informed and the shared approach to decision-making. The former preserves patient autonomy and represents a division of labour where the health care professional provides information on treatment options (including taking no action (Elwyn *et al.* 2000)), benefits and risks. The patient evaluates the information in light of their values, beliefs and life situation and decides which option to pursue. Elwyn *et al.* (2000) refer to informed choice as transferring the responsibility for decision-making. They point out that this can cause patient anxiety when there is uncertainty about what option to pursue and advocate shared decision-making.

Shared decision-making is a two-way process where the health care professional presents the treatment options, benefits and risks, etc., the patient shares their values, beliefs, life situation and perceptions of their illness and the options. These are then discussed and a negotiated way forward is agreed (Charles *et al.* 2003). In other words, the two parties build a consensus (Charles *et al.* 1997). This, too, may not be anxiety-free for either the patient or the nurse as sharing decisions means also sharing uncertainties about the outcome of intervention (Elwyn *et al.* 1999).

Patient partnership and shared decision-making may differ slightly as, although both are more patient-led and bottom-up, Cahill (1996) acknowledges that patient partnership does not necessarily equate with nurse–patient consensus as nurse/patient priorities, etc. may conflict. Patient partnership and shared decision-making are central to the nurse as empowerment facilitator and it is worth noting that Breuera *et al.* (2001) found that as a way of working cancer-care patients more frequently preferred this approach than physicians predicted.

Of the seven key goals identified by the NHS Management Executive (1993) for shifting the balance of power from health care professionals to patients/clients, maximising the availability of information is advanced as the most important factor in empowering patients. To support this the UK Department of Health (2005) has produced an information strategy for long-term neurological conditions to help patients exercise choice.

Undoubtedly, information provision is important but, although they remain unsure of the precise meaning of empowerment, Lovemore and Dann (2002) stress that empowerment is about more than this. Thus, although intervention is underpinned by information (the nurse as informer, see health promotion framework in Chapter 5), the nurse as empowerment facilitator shifts practice away from any information-giving that perpetuates top-down nurse-directed practice based on assessment of need from a professional perspective. Information should be presented in a non-authoritarian way to help enhance patient control (Whitehead and Russell 2004) and not as an adjunct to changing the behaviour of the patient in line with what the nurse deems important or compliance (Piper and Brown 1998a; Kettunen *et al.* 2001).

The nurse as empowerment facilitator is about a patient/client-centred approach operating from a position of 'low social distance' (Beattie 1991: 185) where the patient is at the centre of decision-making (Williams 2002) and the promotion of independence in patients (Faulkner 2001) rather than dependence (Devine 1993). Interventions are grounded in process and empathy, reassurance and support and helping to develop such outcomes as critical awareness (Kettunen *et al.* 2001), confidence and self-esteem, assertiveness and thus bottom-up patient-led decision-making. It is thus concerned with process and outcome (Kettunen *et al.* 2001; Lovemore and Dann 2002).

It represents a biographical model of health where personal issues require review and personal biographies need actively reshaping (Beattie 1993). This is in relation to the patient's experience of bio-psycho-social personal troubles, the symptomatic manifestation of disease and facilitating varying degrees of choice within the patient's pathological biography. The aim is to enhance individual patient control over health and maximise opportunities for choice and self-determination, but within two boundaries. First, the socio-economic context of the patient may have a bearing on choice and decision-making. Second, the treatment decision-making context, for example, emergency care and life-saving intervention, which again might constrain shared decision-making and opportunities for empowerment (Charles *et al*. 1997).

Thus, in summary, while helping to achieve knowledge acquisition and increased understanding (Whitehead and Tones 1991), the nurse as empowerment facilitator seeks to achieve its wider aims essentially by:

- enabling and supporting patients to set their own health promotion agendas and by developing scope for informed choice;
- increasing the patient's ability to understand, cope with, take control of and manage disease and related factors in their lives.

The starting point for this process is acceptance of the patient/client as they are and for whom they are by the nurse (Cartmell and Coles 2000; Williams 2002). It means respecting patient/client autonomy, the right of the latter to make as many of their health care decisions as they choose, and partnership working (Williams 2002). This is about shifting the balance of power in line with Cahill's (1996) nurse–patient partnership, i.e. challenging traditional power relations between the nurse and the patient, equalising the distance between them and developing services around the aspirations and convenience of the latter. It assumes that the nurse is happy to relinquish power and that the patient is prepared to exercise more (Cahill 1996). The UK NMC (2004: 4) refer to partnership working with patients and leave UK nurses, health visitors and midwives in no doubt that they:

> must recognise and respect the role of patients and clients as partners in their care and the contribution they can make to it. This involves identifying their preferences regarding care and respecting these within the limits of professional practice, existing legislation, resources and the goals of the therapeutic relationship.

At the very least, the nurse as empowerment facilitator focuses on patient-defined needs, making sure patients are fully aware of treatment options and their implications, and fosters active patient participation (Williams 2002). Gibson (1991) stresses that patients are capable of making their own health-related decisions, although they may need help and information to do so, and their capacity for personal growth and self-determination must be respected.

Malin and Teasdale (1991) extend this respect for patient autonomy to decision-making related to treatment. This accords with the belief that patients often know best about their individual health, have a right to be involved in all related decisions and that there should be mutual respect between patients and health care professionals (NHSE 1997). There should be the opportunity for carers and family to be involved and there needs to be close communication between all members of the multidisciplinary team (Cartmell and Coles 2000).

Piper (2007b) agrees that providing information about the cause and effect of disease is an important aspect of the nurse as empowerment facilitator, but contends that nurses need to listen rather than just tell. They also need to listen without interrupting (Faulkner 2001), hear what patients are saying and, for example, in relation to pain management engage in active listening (Cartmell and Coles 2000). The Department of Health (2004c) contends that a listening culture requires nurses to:

- encourage patients to express their concerns;
- hear these criticisms;
- treat the above with the seriousness they deserve.

Piper (2007b) goes on to say that it is also not just about acknowledging the desirability of and enabling active patient participation in decisions on clinical matters at any one time, but about ensuring that patients are not only aware of the options open to them but able to exercise informed choice at every opportunity. Facilitating this may mean that nurses have to help patients to tap into and draw on their personal resources and strengths to maximise their autonomy when required and be prepared to act as advocates.

149

Key dimensions of the nurse as empowerment facilitator

Lewin and Piper (2007) summarise the four key dimensions of empowerment identified in the literature (Hogg 1999; Wilkinson and Miers 1999; Kemshall and Littlechild 2000). These are:

- patients' beliefs and ability to have power, influence and control;
- the willingness and commitment of health care professionals to empower patients;
- a perceived change by patients in the power or control over their care;
- equality of opportunity and freedom from discrimination.

Although Lewin and Piper (2007) point to Byrt and Dooher's (2002) suggestion that empowerment is incomplete unless all four dimensions are addressed, Piper and Brown (1998a) emphasise that successful empowerment will depend upon the attitude of the nurse, with Faulkner (2001) advancing the same about disempowerment. Participants in Faulkner's (2001) study of models of interaction between nurses and older patients identified a number of indicators of disempowerment. Patients felt disempowered when nurses spoke to them in patronising tones, i.e. as if they were a child, removed food or drink before it was finished, tried to coerce patients to eat when they didn't want to and ignored patients even when they appeared to know that the patient needed assistance.

Cartmell and Coles (2000) add that cancer patients felt disempowered when in pain, in response to perceived physical changes, by emotional distress and feelings of isolation. To help redress disempowerment in such circumstances it is important, for example when patients are in pain, to respond quickly to alleviate the suffering (Faulkner 2001). Pain assessment/reassessment and opportunity for patients to gain information and ask questions to make informed choices regarding pain management must be built in to the process to help build a trusting relationship. Informed choice extends to type of analgesia and how it is delivered (Cartmell and Coles 2000).

Treating patients as equals, valuing their perceptions and experiences and working to individualised care plans as agreed in partnership with the patient requires empathic understanding and fostering a sense of perceived locus of control (Lovemore and Dann 2002). Intervention needs to be non-hierarchical, non-coercive and a power-sharing therapeutic partnership that minimises the official role of the nurse as a representative of a health care institution (Kettunen *et al.* 2001).

The process is consistent with the development of co-production initiatives in health care. Edgreen (1998) refers to co-production as an approach to cardiac rehabilitation that enables patients, in effect, to be a member of their own health care team by playing an active and significant part in decision-making and in the care process. This might be helped by the use of lay terminology, ward rounds that include the patient and the use of patient-held records (Williams 2002).

However, although the nurse as empowerment facilitator should reflect the patient's perceptions of what is appropriate in terms of health and disease management and possible behaviour change, this does not exclude the nurse from raising an issue. The point is that this must be in a sensitive and non-threatening manner (Piper and Brown 1998a). Hence, the issues may still include smoking-cessation support, stress and weight management.

Zerwkh (1992) identifies a number of strategies used by community public health nurses (PHNs) to foster choice. Consistent with Hopson and Scally (1981) and Tones (2001), empowerment is seen as a process of helping people realise that they have choices and can take charge of their lives. It involves the use of listening skills, giving time to people to allow them to articulate and discuss their needs and the promotion of self-esteem and self-determination. An empowerment strategy includes advocacy, analysing and providing straightforward and candid feedback on the reality of a situation as perceived by the PHN and helping clients reflect on and gain insight into their lives. The PHN also seeks to foster personal responsibility and autonomy among those who deny responsibility and empowerment through a relationship of partnership.

Participants in Piper's (2004) study added that empowerment includes fostering non-judgemental communication and support, sensitivity in relation to social stigma and associated isolation and the promotion of hope. Other important indicators of empowering practice were self-medication (Williams 2002; Piper 2004) and helping patients value themselves and their decisions. As has been seen, then, the nurse as empowerment facilitator is concerned with process and outcome. In other words, it focuses on both the nature of the nurse–patient relationship and the aims, methods and evaluation criteria in the form of impact (intermediate outcome) and outcomes of simple, day-to-day, pragmatic, enabling strategies, as summarised in Table 7.1, and encapsulates empowerment as an applied technology (Tones 2001).

EMPOWERMENT AS A TECHNOLOGY

For Tones (2001), empowerment as an applied technology is a skills-based process focusing on the indicators of practice of the type in Box 7.1. It involves a face-to-face encounter between the health promoter and the patient/client. The first skill required by the former is communicator. Here, the emphasis is on the patient/client's felt needs, information needs, establishing a rapport using listening and counselling skills and providing tailored information via an appropriate medium.

Second, the health promoter should check patient/client motivation levels and facilitate decision-making. Intervention should be concerned to explore their values, attitudes, beliefs and skills and seek to modify beliefs about personal control while taking account of social context. Skills development includes those of a psychomotor (hands-on, for

Table 7.1 The nurse as empowerment facilitator: individual action perspective

Aims	Process	Impact evaluation indicators	Outcomes evaluation indicators
Empowerment	Humanistic, non-hierarchical patient-centred interaction	Health agenda determined, directed and validated by patient with support from nurses	Feelings of control
Adherence	Neutral information provision	• Understanding • Informed patient decision-making • Patient-led decision-making	Self-esteem
Concordance	Stages of change model	• Coping strategies and reduced anxiety • Confidence • Trust	Quality of life
	Advocacy		Feeling supported
	Peer support	Support group accessed	Patient satisfaction
		Complaints	

BOX 7.1 EXAMPLES OF THE SKILLS FOR EMPOWERMENT AS AN APPLIED TECHNOLOGY

- communicator;
- informer;
- rapport builder;
- facilitator of decision-making;
- modifier of beliefs about control;
- advocate for change;
- an awareness about the social context of health.

(Tones 2001)

BOX 7.2 COMMUNICATION CHECKLIST FOR PATIENT EMPOWERMENT IN NURSING

Do you:

- greet the patient;
- introduce yourself and explain who you are, your role and purpose;
- use the patient's name;
- ensure that the patient is comfortable;
- make eye contact with the patient;
- observe and respond to verbal and non-verbal cues;
- focus on, listen to and show an interest in what the patient is saying;
- ask open-ended questions;
- tell the patient that information will be recorded;
- consider the appropriateness and accuracy of your advice;
- summarise what was said and agreed;
- get feedback from the patient;
- thank the patient and bid them farewell?

(after Laverack 2005)

---

example, injection technique) nature, decision-making and other social and life skills. Third, the role of the health promoter is to provide support and help the patient/client develop self-regulating skills, mobilise peer support, act as an advocate for social and environmental change and to monitor progress.

In line with 'communicator' as the first indicator of empowerment as a technology (Tones 2001), Faulkner (2001), the UK Department of Health (2004) and Laverack (2005) also stress the importance of communication as a strategy to help patients/clients gain power. Laverack (2005) advances some pertinent questions for auditing empowering practice, which are slightly modified for nursing in the communication checklist in Box 7.2.

Kettunen *et al.* (2001) outline a range of communication practices that facilitate patient empowerment when preparing for surgery. They include tactfully exploring and encouraging patients to vent their worries about surgery and presenting a positive outcome for the future. They emphasise the importance of the structure of the communication process, i.e. speech formulae, a tentative discussion style and that nurses should pay attention to how patients express themselves and the type of language used. To assist further with a more positive surgical outcome it is important for nurses to:

- give accurate information about forthcoming surgery;
- increase knowledge and understanding about pain and pain management;
- acknowledge the positive elements of patient coping strategies.

(Devine 1993)

Similarly, for shared decision-making Elwyn *et al.* (2000) identified a number of competencies and skills as summarised and modified for use herein in Box 7.3. Empowerment then, is about fostering a relationship based on confidentiality and reciprocal conversation (Kettunen *et al.* 2001). In includes mutual respect and trust and, for Devine (1993), nurses placing their skills and expertise at the disposal of patients.

To be empowered patients need not only relevant information about their illness and care options with nurses checking that the information is understood, but also clear answers to related questions to facilitate informed choice. They may also benefit from using a patient decision aid such as that developed by Sawka *et al.* (1998) for the surgical treatment of early-stage breast cancer. This was produced to help women choose the intervention that they felt most suited their needs given that the options produce the same type of outcome.

In addition, as Parsloe (1997) points out, empowerment is not necessarily an all or nothing concept. It operates along a continuum and it is not always the big issues that are the most important. For example, a care-home resident may not want to be consulted on how the home is managed but may be very concerned to choose what time they go to bed, when to have a cup of tea, etc. (Parsloe 1997).

BOX 7.3 A SUMMARY OF SKILLS AND COMPETENCIES OF SHARED DECISION-MAKING

- providing the opportunity for patients to be involved in all aspects of decision-making;
- clarifying the preferred role of the patient in relation to shared decision-making;
- fully exploring patient fears and expectations;
- exploring the range of treatment options in full;
- identifying the preferred format and provision of patient-specific information;
- checking that the patient understands the information and monitoring their reaction to it;
- enabling patients to make, discuss or defer decisions;
- arranging a follow-up appointment to allow for reconsideration.

(after Elwyn *et al.* 2000)

She suggests that the focus should perhaps be on how to create conditions that enable people to be empowered, and this would require:

155

- a determination on the part of the nurse to understand the patient/client;
- a positive relationship between the nurse and the patient/client;
- self-awareness in the nurse;
- careful use of language;
- an agreement on ways of working.

In line with Laverack (2005, Box 7.2), Parsloe's (1997) empowering conditions would be assisted further by nurses being sensitive and courteous, remembering and recognising patients/clients and speaking to them by name, explaining the reason for any delays and apologising for keeping them waiting (Department of Health 2004c). This not only helps make patients/clients feel important but also facilitates meaningful discussion. Conversely, this is inhibited by impatient, patronising or disrespectful nurses (Department of Health 2004c). Similarly, patients in Faulkner's (2001) study felt that simple interventions by nurses such as allowing patients time to complete tasks, familiarising them with their surroundings, ensuring that they have their call bells within reach and are quiet at night so that patients can sleep, help empower.

EMPOWERMENT AND THE EXPERT PATIENT

The UK Expert Patient programme is seen as a new way to approach and manage chronic disease in the twenty-first century (Department of Health 2001a). The rationale for its inception is that patients with enduring disease often have an advanced understanding of their condition and that this resource, if harnessed, could improve the quality of patients' care and life. Consistent with the literature already referred to, the idea is to move patients away from simply being passive recipients of care toward empowering them to be active decision-makers, to see themselves as partners in their own care and treatment and to accept some responsibility for its management. To help achieve this, patients may have the opportunity to attend a self-management programme to help improve their confidence, resourcefulness and belief that they can be expert patients. The Department of Health (2001a) maintain that research suggests expert patients are more likely to experience a number of tangible benefits such as:

- less severe symptoms (including pain), a more stable disease process and slower deterioration;
- less fatigue, sleep-deprivation and low energy levels and more activity;
- improved resourcefulness, perception of control and fewer emotional problems and thus improved life satisfaction;
- a better quality nurse–patient relationship.

EMPOWERMENT AND ADVOCACY

Advocacy is an acknowledged part of health promotion and thus empowerment, but, as with the latter, it has been variously defined and is representational, facilitative and may involve lobbying (Carlisle 2000). Representational advocacy is where the nurse protects or defends the interests of patients when the patient is unable to, for example because they are feeling too unwell, and should reflect patient-defined needs and aspirations. This may bring the nurse into conflict with fellow professionals and thus is a necessary but not necessarily an easy part of empowering patients. For example, Piper (2004) refers to the role of a breast-care nurse specialist who spends time exploring the needs of the patient. The nurse helps the woman exercise informed choice by, if required, keeping other health care professionals at bay in the short term until the woman is ready, has explored all the options, talked it over with significant others and has made the choice that is right for her.

ADHERENCE AND CONCORDANCE

In Chapter 6 adherence was described as a negotiated and consensual treatment agreement between the health care professional and the patient/client in a spirit of co-operation and partnership (Vermeire *et al.* 2001). It is where the patient commits to a treatment regime that they have actively helped to plan and implement (Elrod 2007). They stick to this agreement (Hobden 2006a) and do not stray from this or use other medication (Ulfvarson *et al.* 2007).

Adherence may be assisted by increasing patient knowledge, effective coping skills in response to bad news, good health care professional–patient/client communication and social support (Eggleston *et al.* 2007). From a practical perspective, Vermeire *et al.* (2001) give examples of adherence-aiding strategies. These include:

- involving patients in the negotiation of treatment objectives and the treatment plan;
- minimising the complexity of the treatment and giving clear explanations;
- tailoring the treatment to the patient's lifestyle;
- use of reminders;
- family support;
- information about side-effects;
- exploring the patient's perceptions, feelings, expectations and understanding about the illness and treatment;
- active listening and empathy;
- monitoring adherence.

The National Aids Manual (1999) suggests examples of reminders to take medication, such as a written daily schedule that can be ticked-off after taking medication, a pillbox with a timer and Medimax or Dosett boxes, which are partitioned containers that contain individual daily medication. Aides-memoire such as refrigerator magnets or stickers may also be useful (Elrod 2007). Possible barriers to adherence are lack of confidence (Elrod 2007), living alone, the use of recreational drugs (Pratt *et al.* 2001), less severe disease, competing life priorities, a lack of time and a fatalistic attitude (Eggleston *et al.* 2007). Failing health, copious medication and a lack of quality information may also play a part (Ulfvarson *et al.* 2007).

Concordance goes further in being more concerned to reflect patient-led/defined outcomes, devolve power to the patient in consultations and improve patient satisfaction (Hobden 2006b). The emphasis is on the quality and experience of the consultation and not on behavioural

157

outcomes, and shared decision-making but with primacy given to the patient's aspirations and choices. The patient perspective and ability to manage their health is acknowledged and respected together with the impact they feel the disease has on their life (Hobden 2006a). Thus, the consultation process should explore the patient perspective, the potential outcome of informed choice when not following the advice of the nurse and seek to achieve mutual understanding while providing non-judgemental support as the patient/client weighs up the relative merits of the options open to them (Hobden 2006b).

HELPING PEOPLE CHANGE

Piper and Brown (1998b) highlight the prominence given to the use of applied health psychology in the form of 'the stages of change model' of Prochaska and DiClemente (1982) in the UK in the 1990s. They note that it formed the conceptual base of a cascade training programme in the UK aimed at, among others, nurses working in primary health care.

Piper and Brown (1998b) would argue that in advancing ways of developing coping strategies (Segan *et al.* 2004) the stages of change model can be used as an integral part of the nurse as empowerment facilitator. However, the caveat is that this should only be when either the patient identifies the need for changing an aspect of health-related behaviour or the nurse raises the issue in a sensitive and non-threatening way. As with any empowerment intervention, the focus should still be on informed choice, developing the decision-making skills of the patient and thus an increase in the perception of patient control and not on behavioural outcomes predetermined by the nurse. Piper and Brown (1998b) emphasise that the focus for the nurse is support, advice and skills-building and that any change in health-related behaviour must be decided and instigated by the patient in their own time.

A full account of the stages of change is beyond the scope of this chapter and the reader is referred to the original authors' (Prochaska and DiClemente 1982) work for a detailed exposition of the process and to Naidoo and Wills (2000). In brief, however, the cycle has four active stages through which people who change successfully move whatever the health-related behaviour. These are preceded by pre-contemplation; where people are not seriously thinking about change, have not made any attempt to do so in the last year (Segan, Borland and Greenwood 2004) and thus are not on the cycle. This gives a total of five stages (Prochaska *et al.* 1992).

The entry point for the cycle is contemplation or preparation (Segan *et al.* 2004). Here, as a result of cognitive dissonance, people become more self-aware about an aspect of their health-related behaviour, for example smoking, and its negative consequences, and think about the positive consequences of change but continue to smoke. Action is when a person has decided to change, for example stop smoking, and maintenance is about strategies to maintain the change. Relapse, an integral part of the cycle, is where, for example, following a stressful life-event the original behaviour is reverted to and the person moves back to the contemplation stage of the cycle or leaves the cycle altogether, i.e. becomes a pre-contemplator not thinking about change. It is not uncommon for individuals to repeat the cycle several times before behaviour change is successful (Prochaska *et al.* 1992).

The transient nature of the nurse–patient relationship means that for most nurses it is unrealistic to think that they would accompany a patient through the entire cycle of change. The cycle is highlighted as nurses need to have an understanding of the process to enable them to provide stage-specific support for those patients/clients engaging in health-related behaviour change.

Nurses also need to understand the following about the cycle. First, that poor patient/client motivation, defensiveness, resistance to change and limited interpersonal skills together with inadequate skills of the health care professional undermine the change process (Prochaska *et al.* 1992). Second, and while rebutted by DiClemente (2005), the stages of change is not without its critics. For example, Segan *et al.* (2004) contend that there is a lack of evidence supporting its claims and West (2005) criticises the arbitrary dividing lines between the stages, the assumption that patients/clients make logical, well-balanced plans, and doubts its value beyond common sense.

159

EMPOWERMENT AS HUMANISTIC MEDICAL MODEL HEALTH PROMOTION

The nurse as empowerment facilitator perpetuates the view that interventions by nurses can develop and enhance personal patient power (Gilbert 1995). However, it is important to remember that intervention cannot be divorced from the reality of political and professional power relations (Skelton 1994) or ideology. Beattie (1993) aligns empowerment with the culture of individualism and socio-political and socio-cultural perspective of Douglas (1982). This has a stance of minimal social structure and control, an emphasis on the private domain and intervention for personal development. Health promotion of this nature is 'libertarian', 'anti-collective' (Beattie 1991: 184) and anti-authoritarian based on a humanistic philosophy of self-help.

Thus, the nurse as empowerment facilitator translates into what Gomm (1993) refers to as a helping relationship rather than one concerned with patient/client emancipation and it can be argued that it is misleading to depict it as a relationship of equals. For example, for the most part where choice is facilitated the focus is on sharing therapeutic possibilities and helping patients make the best use of available resources and options. Any change in the dynamic of the nurse–patient relationship is a modification of enduring and traditional roles. Although the use of power may be attenuated, the hierarchical culture and context of practice and the expertise gap between professional and patient, albeit exercised in line with codes of professional practice, help preserve disparity. Thus, while similar to what Jack (1995a) describes as enablement, empowerment here differs in helping patients to gain some control and influence over their experience and their use of health services within, but not beyond the professional and ideological context of the medical model.

This may also apply to contemporary aspects of practice such as adherence and concordance. For example, when Rosen *et al.* (2007) suggest that for HIV-positive patients struggling with adhering to their antiretroviral therapy regime intervention may need to be more intensive and use contingency-management counselling and monetary reward, the difference between compliance and adherence may lack some clarity. Indeed Lovemore and Dann (2002) go so far as to suggest that concordance can be viewed as simply a new tactic for managing non-compliant patients/clients and a sop to those who demand to be consulted.

Face-to-face-type interventions to empower by nurses take place within the spaces allowed by the medical model and its associated institutional structures. Hence, empowerment may be constrained by the philosophy, organisation and delivery of care (Latter 1998; Salmon and Hall 2004). These processes and structures are both a product and an agent and create systems of power within which nurses practise. It does not involve giving over power to the enabled and in not challenging the unequal social structure acts as a form of social control reinforcing the social and political status quo (Jack 1995a).

In part, this is consistent with Gott and O'Brien (1990b) who found that facilitation, enablement and empowerment were interpreted as traditional top-down and nurse-led information-giving interventions emphasising risk management and prevention in relation to disease.

For some, then, empowerment represents a relatively straightforward set of skills-based interventions for nurses. For others empowerment, in focusing on professionally ratified personal development, represents professional imperialism (Jack 1995b), social control via self-regulation (Rose 1996), and an extension of the victim-blaming stance (Beattie 1991) and thus a means of perpetuating inequalities in power.

Although there is now an expectation that nurses will encourage patients to take control of their illness or treatments (Salmon and Hall 2004), McEwan and Bhopal (1991) are sceptical and believe that the unstated objective of self-empowerment is behaviour change in the direction health promoters prefer. Piper and Brown (1998b) add that nurses may espouse empowerment principles and adopt models such as the stages of change (Prochaska and DiClemente 1982; Naidoo and Wills 2000) ostensibly to facilitate change. In practice this may translate into nurses masquerading as empowerment champions by using their understanding of theory to induce predetermined behavioural outcomes, for example, stopping smoking or eating a weight-reducing diet. In pursuing a nursing and medical model agenda they would be contradicting empowerment principles by undermining patient control and the patient-directed philosophy of the nurse as empowerment facilitator.

Salmon and Hall (2004) go further by contending that when nurses adopt strategies in practice or merely use the language of empowerment they are helping to redefine boundaries of nursing responsibility. In empowering patients and devolving decision-making, etc., nurses are reducing their own levels of responsibility for them. They see it as part of wider political and cultural change where an emphasis on individual autonomy and rights is actually allowing state institutions to reduce their level of responsibility for individuals. They suggest that the imposition of empowerment on patients may actually undermine their interests. There is also the potential for it to be used as a substitute for service (Parsloe 1997).

Salmon and Hall (2004) also observe that the literature suggests that some patients are less than enthusiastic about empowerment. This accords with Lewin and Piper (2007). Although by no means necessarily generalisable to other populations due to the small number of participants in the study, the particular critical-care clinical milieu, etc., nevertheless their findings make interesting reading. The exploratory, small-scale study investigated coronary-care patients' perceptions of empowerment and strengthening patient choice. They found that the empowerment agenda, i.e. the right of patients to be primary decision-makers and directors of their treatment and care were a low priority. Most of the patients in the study were happy to devolve these decisions to nurses and other health care professionals based on the confidence they had in their expertise. In summary, patients were well satisfied with their care, and their individual empowerment was of peripheral concern with decision-making readily abdicated when experiencing acute illness. In relation to the latter, the desire to be empowered may not be a constant state but a dynamic one waxing and waning in tandem with the severity of the illness (Cahill 1996).

Similarly, although Loft *et al.* (2003) found that the nurse–patient relationship was disempowering, this was not the major issue for the participants in the study who were more concerned to recover their independence after hip and knee replacement. Their small sample of elderly patients were deferential to the traditional medical model, did not expect an empowering style of interaction between themselves and nurses and did not covet this type of relationship. Thus, the desire for empowerment may not be universal and the assumption that everyone wants to be empowered may be false. Some patients may wish to adopt a passive role and opt to devolve responsibility for decision-making to health care professionals (Henwood *et al.* 2003). An increase in patient rights brings with it an increase in patient responsibilities. Although some health care professionals may feel this is the way forward some patients are still to be convinced (Henwood *et al.* 2003) and some may experience greater anxiety (Elwyn *et al.* 2000).

It may also be too simplistic to assume that the power imbalance can be redressed by, for example, nurses endeavouring to hand over their power to patients (Hewitt-Taylor 2005) as this overlooks the complexity and context of the relationship. In addition, the notion of empowerment may both be engendering false perceptions of democracy because of the imbalance in expertise and contradicting the current medical model ideology of evidence-based practice (McQueen *et al.* 2002). Rather than compatible concepts, evidence-based medicine and empowerment represent a clash of ideologies (Salmon and Hall 2004).

Finally, opportunity-cost further complicates empowerment. The choice of one patient may be for expensive treatment or for treatment that is in limited supply and this may compromise the choice of other patients (Hewitt-Taylor 2004). The same applies to time. Nursing time is limited and costly and copious time spent with one patient may reduce that available for others. To deny this denies the reality of health-care rationing (Hewitt-Taylor 2004).

EMPOWERMENT AS 'NEW NURSING'

The empowerment in nursing described in this chapter accords with what Salvage (1990: 42) refers to as a wider and contemporary ideology and 'new nursing' practice. 'New nursing' adopts both a problem-solving and evidence-based approach and a holistic means of intervention. Patients are encouraged to be active partners in care and to exercise informed choice, and the traditional medical model form of nurse–patient relationship is rejected (Salvage 1990). It requires nurses to accept that the decisions patients make may not be consistent with their views and that patients may even reject the help offered by the nurse. It involves nurses surrendering power and control and shifting practice to a position of facilitation and a commitment to serve patient-defined needs rather than that of nurse-led service provision.

CONCLUSION

This chapter has presented a brief theoretical analysis of the nature, purpose, methodologies and intended health gain of the individually focused, process-orientated and humanistically inspired nurse as empowerment facilitator. The focus has been on patient control over health and health-related decision-making and pragmatic enabling strategies for empowerment as an applied technology (Tones 2001) in line with the developing consumer culture in health care.

It can be concluded that it is important to be cognisant of two factors. First, that empowerment is not an all-or-nothing concept and can be enabled at different levels (Parsloe 1997). Second, that caution must be exercised as it should not be assumed that patients/clients are free to change and choose at liberty their health-related behaviour, even if they so desire, as such decisions are influenced by a range of variables. These include social and disease context, financial circumstances and a medical model framework and set of professionally imposed boundaries, etc. However, where possible, the nurse as empowerment facilitator should be adopted by nurses as the more valid individual-action perspective (Piper and Brown 1998a). The process may be helped, as Piper and Brown (1998a) suggest, by nurses reflecting on their empowering practice by asking themselves the slightly modified questions posed by Mitchell (1982) in the empowerment checklist in Box 7.4.

BOX 7.4 PATIENT EMPOWERMENT CHECKLIST

Am I:

- trying to make patients feel inadequate or helping them take control over their health/disease?
- helping patients understand their disease, diagnosis and prognosis or am I mystifying them?
- listening to patients feelings and perceptions of their life-experience and illness and helping them identify and find solutions to the problems they face?
- helping patients to understand the socio-economic and political determinants of illness and disease?

(after Piper and Brown 1998a and Mitchell 1982)

LEARNING TRIGGERS

Having read Chapter 7, complete the learning triggers below to reinforce your understanding of the concepts that have been discussed:

- Define empowerment and empowerment as a technology.
- Summarise the key features of the individual-action perspective the nurse as empowerment facilitator health promotion model.
- List examples of the aims, processes, impact and evaluation criteria and outcomes of intervention.
- Define and differentiate between adherence and concordance.
- Define and differentiate between patient involvement, participation, partnership and shared decision-making.
- Define empowerment and advocacy.
- Summarise the 'helping people change' model of practice.
- Identify the key features of empowerment as humanistic medical-model health promotion.
- Describe how empowerment fits with the concept of 'new nursing'.
- Audit your empowerment practice by asking of yourself and thus of your style of nursing the questions posed in Box 7.2 and Box 7.4.

THE NURSE AS EMPOWERMENT FACILITATOR

8

COMMUNITY ACTION PERSPECTIVE

INTRODUCTION

This chapter is concerned with the concept of the nurse as empowerment facilitator from a community-action perspective and thus health as a social product. As with the nurse as empowerment facilitator from an individual-action perspective, the focus is on process as much as on outcome and a bottom-up locus of control but, as can be seen in the health promotion framework in Chapter 5, on micro population interventions. Intervention is concerned to facilitate a community-led agenda and nurse–community partnership-based practice for collective health gain. A number of ways of working under the auspices of community development aiming to build social capital and capacity, together with community advocacy emanating from a radical humanistic premise and associated socio-political values, are discussed. The chapter also focuses on indicators and practical (i.e. not ideological/theoretical) examples of the health promotion aims, processes, impact and evaluation criteria and outcomes of this contemporary model of 'new' public health practice for nurses, to demonstrate the theory–practice relationship and help bridge this gap.

COMMUNITY

For Green and Kreuter (1990), the community is the central focus for health promotion. However, the meaning of the term community depends on the context in which it is being used (Royal College of Nursing 2002) i.e. who the community is (Laverack and Wallerstein 2001). Allender and Spradley (2005) identify the following three key contexts as relevant to community nursing:

- geographic
- common interest
- health problem.

They point out that a geographic community in the sense of a geographic location can mean a city, town or neighbourhood. It depends upon the size of the population and is more likely to refer to town or county in a low-population area and a school, workplace or neighbourhood in more urban environments (Green and Kreuter 1990). Thus, it is important to clarify that, for the purpose of this chapter and book, community as a geographical location means neighbourhood comprising institutions, a social system and some level of interaction. It assumes at the very least a degree of collective identity, a sense of belonging and shared values, norms and concerns and links and communication via formal and informal networks as per examples in Box 8.1 (Allender and Spradley 2005).

Common interest community refers to groups of people who, rather than sharing a physical environment, have some other important feature of their life in common. They may share a collective social identity, for example, the gay community (Royal College of Nursing 2002; Tones and Green 2004; Allender and Spradley 2005) or professional identity (Tones and Green 2004). Health problem refers to those who share a diagnosis, such as the diabetic community or the HIV-positive community (Allender and Spradley 2005) but may be referred to as community coalition when focusing on, for example, HIV prevention (Mayer *et al.* 1998).

COMMUNITY EMPOWERMENT

The *Ottawa Charter* (WHO 1986) refers to community empowerment as the heart of health promotion. It is a social action process where the community gain power via control and ownership of local groups, organisations and institutions and thus power over their lives and health experience (WHO 1986; Wallerstein and Bernstein 1998). The assumption is that there is an inequality in power or a pressing social problem (Rissel 1994) and that the social and political changes needed to redress powerlessness can only be achieved through active group and community organisation and mobilisation (Laverack and

---

BOX 8.1 EXAMPLES OF COMMUNITY COMMUNICATION AND NETWORK-BUILDING CONDUITS

- schools
- health centres
- churches
- housing associations
- shops
- library
- local newspaper
- gossip.

Wallerstein 2001). An empowered community comprises individuals who feel personally empowered and this, together with collective action for change and control over local resources engenders community empowerment (Rissel 1994).

Thus, Wallerstein and Bernstein (1998) and Rissel (1994) stress that although community empowerment is distinct from individual/ psychological empowerment concerned with enhancing self-esteem and self-efficacy (Wallerstein and Bernstein 1998), active community-member participation and political action does include a psychological element (Rissel 1994). It is also not about individuals having power over others but about realising collective power and taking action to effect community connectedness and change to benefit the community and deliver outcomes, such as an improved quality of life and social justice (Wallerstein and Bernstein 1998).

Wallerstein and Bernstein (1998) draw on Paulo Freire's work, which advocated getting groups to identify and critically assess their problems and develop strategies to overcome these and achieve their goals via empowering education using a three-stage method of:

1 listening: to understand the felt needs of the community and continuing to listen beyond the needs-assessment stage;
2 participatory dialogue: because it might not be possible to solve immediately the problems identified and expressed by a community during participatory dialogue this process involves problem-posing rather than problem-solving;
3 action: to effect change in line with felt needs and the outcomes of the participatory dialogue.

The need for listening is illustrated by Labonte (1989) when he talks about a group of single mothers identifying healthy eating and nutrition as a health need but not from the perspective of cooking on a low budget. Their concern was with the high cost of food and rents, low benefit payments and access to fresh food. Their strategy to address this included a community garden, community meals and exploring the feasibility of setting up a food co-operative (Labonte 1989).

The concerns of community members identified in Snee's (1991) study of neighbourhood needs may also be outside the frame of reference of some nurses. They included poor access to local doctors, the absence of a local chemist, heating costs, the absence of good local food shops, inadequate play facilities for children, inadequate street lighting, traffic congestion, litter, stray dogs and dog excrement.

For Laverack and Wallerstein (2001), the implementation and measurement of community empowerment are difficult processes, while Rissel (1994) cautions that even if community empowerment is demonstrably realised it should not be assumed that it is transferable from one issue to another. He suggests that it may be specific to a topic, i.e. a group may achieve empowerment in one aspect of community life but this may not apply to another. Rissel (1994) adds that there may be degrees of community empowerment and that what can be achieved may depend on the issue. Thus, the greater number of issues over which the community has control the more empowered they are likely to be, and this is a key successful-outcome evaluation indicator. The process requires a facilitative rather than a directive approach by health care professionals to help achieve this outcome (Rissel 1994; Laverack and Wallerstein 2001), which should also be an empowering experience for community members helping them gain power via exercising collectively their personal power (Laverack and Wallerstein 2001).

COMMUNITY CONSULTATION, INVOLVEMENT, PARTICIPATION AND COLLABORATION

As with individual empowerment, the use of terminology associated with community empowerment needs careful consideration and clarification due to the contrasting use of terminology. From his reading of the pertinent literature, Labonte (1993) is careful to distinguish between community consultation, involvement, participation and collaboration. With the former, dialogue starts and stops simply at the level of collecting information from community members as the issue and desired outcome are predetermined. For Labonte (1993), dialogue goes further with community involvement but does not involve power sharing, whereas Handsley (2007a) links it with consultation and participation.

Community participation involves negotiation and shared decision-making in relation to needs assessment, leadership, organisation, resource mobilisation and management, but the extent of community empowerment depends upon how much professional power, negotiated power or community power is exercised. It embraces a philosophy of partnership working, i.e. bringing together members of the community and a multidisciplinary team of health and social care professionals to solve health and social problems (Royal College of Nursing 2002).

Effective partnership working requires community members to be established in their locality, to be accountable to a constituency and for nurses to engage with their agenda without trying to push the strategic objectives and targets of the health or social care institution they represent (Labonte 1993). To achieve this, Raphael *et al.* (1999) recommend using a collaborative, participatory or community-controlled approach to identifying community needs and strengths within nine quality-of-life domains, including establishing the extent to which community members have a sense of physical, social and community belonging.

However, Laverack and Wallerstein (2001) contend that whereas community empowerment is concerned with socio-political change, liberation and activism for the acquisition of community power, a community participation approach may not seek any of these outcomes. Participation in a programme may build capacity and skills but may not deliver power to the community. It is also important to note that partnership working can also be used to emphasise partnership between professional agencies and working across organisational boundaries on joint community health programmes. The objectives are more concerned with better service co-ordination and delivery, economies of scale and related outcomes (Health Development Agency 2003) than partnership between the community and health and social care professionals.

Collaboration then goes that bit further. It is as for participation but gives greater recognition to the interdependence of stakeholders. Conflict is dealt with constructively, there is collective ownership and responsibility for defining and posing agreed problems, decision-making and managing the process, which is acknowledged as dynamic and evolving (Labonte 1993).

Arnstein's (1969) seminal 'ladder of citizen participation' states that participation is *the* term to use but warns that without the redistribution of power it is a meaningless and frustrating ritual. As with Carey's (2000) participation spectrum the ladder is a hierarchical continuum of community empowerment/disempowerment. It contains the three categories of non-community participation, token community participation and degrees of community empowerment representing gradations of power, as can be seen in the version of the ladder modified for nursing in Figure 8.1.

The manipulation and therapy of non-participation fits with the medical-model ideology and processes of the nurse as behaviour change agent approach (Chapter 6) to health promotion. It is only concerned to tick the community participation box, i.e. create an illusion that the community has been involved in the planning or managing of programmes. It promotes a top-down agenda of professionally

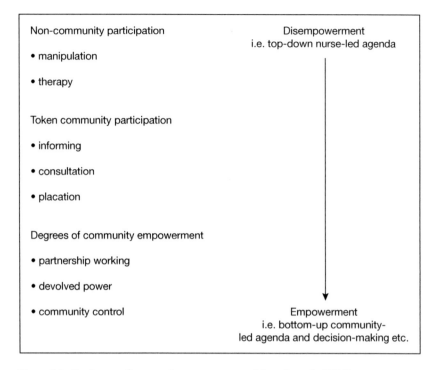

Figure 8.1 Continuum of community empowerment (after Arnstein 1969)

determined social issues and encourages community members to adopt mainstream social values and behaviours.

The informing, consultation and placation of token community participation that allows the community a voice and the potential for a small measure of influence is similar to Labonte's (1993) community consultation with the power of decision-making, etc., still resting firmly with existing powerholders outside of the community. Nevertheless, for Arnstein (1969) informing people about their rights and choices and consulting them about issues are important first steps toward community empowerment as long as the process is not undermined by one-way, top-down and evasive communication. The degrees of community empowerment categories are the start of real community empowerment and range from partnership working and negotiated outcomes to the delegation of full power and community control (Arnstein 1969).

Carey (2000) talks more simply about levels of participation ranging from low to high with corresponding action by community members. Movement along the spectrum brings an increase in dialogue and negotiation ultimately leading to nurses and agencies becoming a resource rather than strategic decision-makers and programme drivers. The extreme end of low participation actually means no participation and no community consultation, this progresses to top-down, one-way information-giving to a passive and compliant community and consultation that canvasses support for professionally led intervention. The 'advises' category remains professionally led but allows for community members to comment on proposals before moving to a position of 'authority', i.e. involvement in planning with health and social care professionals and culminates in community control and thus the highest point of community participation.

It may be that the extent of community participation is indicative of the power the community holds. Therefore, there is the potential to use community participation as a strategy to help increase the perception of power among community members and that through collective action they can resolve their problems and improve health experience while acquiring skills (David *et al.* 1998).

The *Liverpool Declaration on the Right to Health* (1988) states that health for all requires participation by all and ensuring that the community have a say in decision-making on health issues. For this to happen, and for effective community participation, David *et al.* (1998) advance a number of prerequisites that need to be in place. These include a political climate and policy and legislation, health service and health care professional context conducive to decentralisation and meaningful participation. Experience of inter-agency partnership working, a community that is interested in health and related issues, prepared to participate and accept responsibility and effective community communication channels are also needed.

COMMUNITY DEVELOPMENT

The UK Royal College of Nursing (2002) equates community development for nurses working to improve public health with community participation. It is about facilitating health gain via bottom-up, community-led identification, assessment and articulation of shared health and social needs and priorities and helping to find and implement solutions acceptable to and owned by the community (Labonte 1993; Royal College of Nursing 2002; Gilchrist 2007; Smithies and Webster undated). Community development starts at the community's point of reference and they set the pace (Dinham 2005). While reflecting a community (as opposed to a top-down professionally prescribed) agenda based on subjective community perceptions and local knowledge (Smithies and Webster undated) it can include tackling health determinants and inequalities rather than just responding to their consequences (Watkins and Wilson 1997; Department of Health 2001b).

Community development is a holistic approach that, in addressing health and related social issues, goes beyond medical model individual 'risk factors' and health-related behaviour and is intervention by professionals to help communities to help themselves (Gilchrist 2007). It requires public health nurses to adopt Smithies and Webster's (undated) inclusive ways of working, i.e. enabling community members from all sections of the community to be the key decision-makers and central to all stages of planning and delivering intervention. For this to happen, access to resources and services, professional boundaries, organisations and structures and democratic processes need to be opened up and management structures decentralised (*Liverpool Declaration on the Right to Health* 1988; Smithies and Webster undated). For local democracy to work community service providers need to work democratically and be transparent and accountable (Hashagen and Paxton 2007).

Community development is about enabling community members to work together to build their own understanding and recognition of what can be achieved while strengthening local democracy (Webster 1989). For Webster (1989), communities need to be organised so that they can articulate and action their agendas and inform and influence local health policy and service delivery. Community development objectives include encouraging self and mutual help, raising political consciousness and lobbying for change via pressure groups. The essence is to achieve change with the community members at the hub of the process (Croft and Beresford 1992).

Thus, Webster (1989) outlines four elements of community development work:

- helping the community to establish support groups on topics they feel are important and contribute to service planning for intervention to improve health;
- facilitating access both to places in which to hold community/group meetings and activities, and finance for community activity and projects;
- facilitating the setting up of a network for information exchange and an infrastructure for training, skills and evaluation strategy development;
- helping to develop a strategy for community (neighbourhood) and interest-group participation to inform and influence local health policy and service delivery.

These elements require the negotiation of goals and methods with community members to build an inclusive consensus (Shediac-Rizkallah and Bone 1998; Dinham 2005) to help sustain community development projects (Shediac-Rizkallah and Bone 1998). This should be accompanied by combining professional and community-determined indicators to evaluate community development projects (Dixon and Sindall 1994).

CAPACITY BUILDING AND SOCIAL CAPITAL

Public health nurses also need to adopt Smithies and Webster's (un-dated) inclusive ways of working because the process, i.e. building local capacity for social capital is as important as the outcomes of intervention. Capacity building is about developing the ability of a community to initiate change (Handsley 2007a). It is used herein to refer to related community empowerment processes but it is important to note that as with all the related concepts it can be used in other ways. For example, capacity building was defined by the focus group participants in Hawe *et al.*'s (1998) study as developing the health promotion and problem-solving skills and resources at the five levels of individuals, health care teams and organisations, across organisa-tions and within the community. Thus, it is also used to describe health infrastructure, i.e. the capacity of local health and social care services to deliver, maintain and sustain programs and the capacity of organisations and communities to problem-solve (Hawe *et al.* 1998).

Crisp *et al.* (2000) similarly outline the four main approaches to capacity building of top-down and bottom-up organisational approaches focusing on agency policies and practices, and skills development of staff respectively, partnership working to strengthen the relationships between agencies, and community organising involving community members. They stress that evaluating the latter must focus on organisation and community process indicators (Crisp *et al.* 2000) and not individual outcomes.

In the US the National Academy of Sciences (2002) also call for agencies to build better partnerships both with each other and with community organisations and for the community to lead the identifi-cation of health needs and evaluation of outcomes for community health gain and reduction in inequalities. They contend that public health departments should assist this process by providing access to technical support and resources, emphasising the need to continue to engage the community and maintain community leadership and to institutionalise positive project outcomes in the community or health care system.

Engaging with communities and catalysing local action may help build and strengthen social cohesion, trust and capacity, i.e. develop social organisations, civic participation, social reciprocity and co-operation for mutual benefit creating an unseen glue binding people and communities together leading to social capital (Kawachi *et al.* 1997). Whereas for Morrow (1999) it is something of a contested and vague concept with various meanings, a community with a high level of social capital indicators as described above, i.e. strong com-munication and social support networks, etc., is also likely to be one that is cohesive (Cooper *et al.* 1999).

Kawachi *et al.* (1997), Cooper *et al.* (1999) and Gilchrist (2007) point to a growing body of evidence linking the quality of personal relationships and companionship, social networks and connectedness, i.e. social capital to real and perceived positive health gain. Social capital can be defined as the social, economic and cultural resources of a community. The greater the resource-base the higher the potential for social capital via collective action on local problems and support for community members when needed (Cooper *et al.* 1999).

Cooper *et al.*'s (1999) review and analysis of British data for the UK Health Education Authority refers to findings on social capital acting as a stress buffer protecting people from stress or helping them manage it more effectively. Stress is reportedly higher in individuals who feel depressed, socially isolated or that lack social support. High levels of social capital helps to increase tolerance and empathy, reduce cynicism and helps people to cope better with social pressures (Putnam 2000). Interpersonal interactions associated with group and community membership and identity and the feeling of solidarity with those with similar life experience(s) are also advanced as helping to prevent (Gilchrist 2007) and fight physical and mental illness (Putnam 2000) and maintain physical health (Cooper *et al.* 1999).

The bigger the social network the better as this enables more access to meaningful social relationships, supports self esteem (Cooper *et al.* 1999) and delivers more potential positive health outcomes. It may also be that maximum health gain accrues from having social support during stressful times provided by people from the same generation, gender, ethnic group and social class and thus with shared life-experiences (Cooper *et al.* 1999). They also note from the research that:

- those in married relationships enjoy lower levels of mortality than the unmarried and socially isolated;
- the impact of widowhood is greater on men than women as often their wife provides their only link to a social network;
- social network size tends to decrease as people get older.

Gilchrist (2007) cites Granevtter's (1973) reference to strong and weak ties to help define further social capital. The former refers to relationships that have a deep emotional connection and the latter to where there is a social connection but not of the same depth or emotional significance. Putnam (2000) similarly refers to bonding and bridging as two important distinctions of social capital. The definitions below are slightly modified to serve the purpose of the nurse as empowerment facilitator from a community/collective-action perspective while remaining true to the spirit of the originals:

- Bonding – close, long-standing, committed relationships, e.g. friends, family, close work colleagues, immediate neighbours.
- Bridging – looser connections but overlapping interests/commitments. For example, relationships with members of the wider geographical community, professional networks beyond immediate work colleagues and locality and social groups beyond the local neighbourhood.

Community development seeks to build social capital mostly through bridging and linking, i.e. establishing relationships between community groups (Gilchrist 2007) and, in this case, between these and public health nurses.

PRAGMATIC COMMUNITY EMPOWERMENT STRATEGIES FOR NURSES

Public health nursing operates along a continuum of individual- to population-based interventions for bio-psycho-social health gain (Elliston and Wilkinson 2004) and across socio-economic and demographic groups. However, the nurse as empowerment facilitator from a collective-action perspective is concerned with the process and outcome of the nurse–community relationship. The aims, methods and evaluation criteria in the form of impact (intermediate outcome) and outcomes of community empowerment, social capital and capacity building are summarised in Table 8.1.

Nevertheless, as with individual empowerment, the nurse as empowerment facilitator from a collective-action perspective also embraces the role of the nurse as informer (see health promotion framework in Chapter 5) while similarly shunning top-down, nurse-directed practice based on assessment of need from a professional perspective. Information should be presented in a non-authoritarian way and is for helping communities to make choices and access services (Department of Health 2006a) they deem appropriate to their

PRACTICE

Table 8.1 The nurse as empowerment facilitator: community-action perspective

Aims	Process	Impact evaluation indicators	Outcome evaluation indicators
Community empowerment	Radical humanist, non-hierarchical community-centred interaction	Health agenda determined, directed and validated by community with support from nurses	Quality of life
Social capital		• Community-led needs assessment	Social justice
Capacity building	Community development 'community consultation' 'community involvement' 'community participation' 'community collaboration'	• Community leadership, e.g. decision-making • Community coping strategies • Feelings of confidence, community trust and connectedness • Network of community relationships	Community control of resources
	'listening' 'participatory dialogue'		
	(see text for references for above)		

needs, to access budget holders, those in positions of civic power, education, training and skills development programs, etc.

Public health nurses need to start the process of helping to build or develop further capacity via greater civic participation for social capital and community development within local communities in three key ways. First, nurses with a public health remit must find out about the socio-cultural dynamics of local groups and the community; what makes it tick (Royal College of Nursing 2002; Handsley 2007b). The health and social needs and priorities must be defined by community members and reflected in community development projects (Handsley 2007c; Mittelmark 2007) and local health service commissioning and provision (Department of Health 2006a). It should be a systematic and rigorous process and include the views of those difficult to reach who may have the greatest needs but who are often not heard (Department of Health 2006a).

This might mean working with local communities to help them identify and target the health needs of particular neighbourhoods or the socially isolated. Examples include the elderly or the homeless (Department of Health 1999a, 2001b), social inclusion issues such as integrating excluded refugees (Hamer and Easton 2002) and supporting young, vulnerable single mothers by facilitating the setting up of a support group (Department of Health 1999a). Helping to enable greater participation in the identification of local need could involve public health nurses in collective research with members of the community for developing strategies to enhance health (Cork 1990). The findings may translate into helping to establish a community resource base and infrastructure on a diverse range of issues. Although these might be focused on finance via credit unions or the physical environment (Hamer and Easton 2002) or a more traditional medical model agenda, they may identify the need for wide ranging but distinct social health-focused projects such as:

- fruit and vegetable co-operatives
- community cafes
- support groups
- crèche co-operatives
- cook and taste sessions
- tenants' groups
- community newspapers
- women's support groups.

(Watkins and Wilson 1997: 45)

Second, and as a way-in to working with a community, public health nurses need to identify and cultivate relationships with community leaders, gatekeepers and those that chair local groups, etc. In tandem with this it is important to make contact with potential influential allies such as health service managers, non-statutory organisations, local politicians and members of parliament (Royal College of Nursing 2002) who the community may want to access. Decision-makers could also be accessed by sitting on, or by submitting verbal and written evidence to service provider committees, multi-agency working groups and healthy alliances.

Third, public health nurses may be involved in facilitating the development of new skills and social roles over a sustained period, which may be a hit-and-miss experience for the community members (Frankish and Green 1994). During this process the challenges are to establish who legitimately represents the community and engage the disinterested and those who prefer decisions to be made by health care professionals (David *et al.* 1998). There are also the challenges of mediating between different interest groups or those with competing agendas and of ensuring that community development practice is in line with the robust and inclusive principles in Box 8.2 (Department of Health 2001b: 28). These principles can function, in effect, as a partial code of practice.

Community development processes do not tend to happen spontaneously (Gilchrist 2007) and, in summary, Hawe *et al.* (1998)

BOX 8.2 COMMUNITY DEVELOPMENT PRINCIPLES

- Participation: everyone having a say in what is right for them in their community.
- Collaboration and partnership: recognising the interdependence of local community structures to improve community health.
- Equality and equity: the belief that people have the right to equal access to resources for the maintenance and promotion of health, and where none exist that they be provided.
- Collective action: bringing people together to deal with issues and needs that they have defined as problematic.
- Empowerment: by which people, organisations and communities gain control over their lives.

(Department of Health 2001b: 28)

found that working for social capital involves engaging the community and challenging thought processes. It is important to respond to the expressed needs and issues of the community, use appropriate language, build local skills and networks and provide incentives for community activity such as financial grants. Health and social care professional and community workers also need to take a back seat and allow others to get the credit and recognition for local initiatives.

Working in this way requires both a recasting (Snee 1991) of the role of public health nurses and a concomitant change in health service management outlook. The latter need to be supportive and understand the long-term nature of community development work, that it involves risk, long-term funding and access to a budget, staff training and a fully accessible public health department (Watkins and Wilson 1997).

To help illustrate pragmatically how hospital nurses might also use the nurse as empowerment facilitator from a community/collective action perspective in a limited way, Piper (2007b) applies the processes to emergency nursing practice. Although a limited part of an emergency nurse's repertoire of health promotion interventions, this way of working can help patients to access and develop social networks and social capital albeit specifically in relation to injury and disease. Emergency nurses can develop directories of national and local self-help and support groups and key contacts for their departments so that patients and significant others can be directed towards these. The virtue of these groups is in helping to reduce isolation; enabling patients and/or their significant others to use their collective resources to determine their common needs, shape their agenda for health, and build support and education networks. Group members can share experiences, help each other develop coping strategies and draw strength from mutual support. They can also challenge the medical and nursing professions and lobby for change in health and social care provision and other local facilities.

In a similar vein, Latter (2001) highlights the potential for hospital nurses to pursue more community-focused health promotion interventions. She gives the examples of a senior nurse on a neuro-muscular ward liaising with a local support group, and suggests liaison and collaboration with community agencies, developing alliances, and deepening and strengthening relationships with wider community health promotion initiatives. Community nurses and midwives can also fulfil this type of role and together with other health and social care professionals can help facilitate and support the setting-up of self-help groups in response to identified need and publicise their existence, purpose and role.

Stewart (1989) advances that mutual-aid self-help groups are important vehicles for health promotion. She suggests that nurses could lead multidisciplinary teams that include self-help group members in planning, implementing and evaluating formal and informal services. They could also assist self-help groups in getting nurses to serve as temporary consultants, speakers and board members in response to invitations from these forums. School nurses could help develop multidisciplinary partnerships with teachers and other interested parties (Department of Health 1999a), including parents and children, for improving school health, and work with pressure groups such as Parents Against Tobacco or community mothers on issues such as safe play areas for children.

COLLECTIVE PATIENT ADVOCACY

Finally, a deviant/paradigm case in Piper's (2004) study generated the concept of the nurse as patient advocate as an aspect of the nurse as empowerment facilitator from a collective-action perspective. Intervention is not with patients on their individual health needs but is an indirect form of practice where the nurse advocates on behalf of a client group. In the study, the nurse was seeking to increase funding and service provision, overcome organisational constraints, promote equal opportunities and place the needs of a particular client group onto the agenda of other health care staff through lobbying, acting as a change agent and an awareness raiser. It is acknowledged that this does not reflect the nurse as empowerment facilitator in the sense of non-directive intervention with members of a geographical community on mutual problems, developing strategies for change independently of social structures and institutions for health gain or engaging in civil protest fighting for social justice. But it is concerned with empowerment on an institutional scale and reflects interventions that are patient/client-centred and symmetric.

SOCIO-POLITICAL AND IDEOLOGICAL FOUNDATIONS AND CRITIQUE

The nurse as empowerment facilitator from a community/collective-action perspective fits conceptually and ideologically with Beattie's (1991) Community Development for Health (CDH). Its socio-political and ideological foundations and processes are those of radical pluralism and communitarian health (Beattie 1993). As with the nurse as empowerment facilitator from an individual-action perspective, in championing participation by autonomous social groups and agitating for social change the practitioner maintains a 'low social distance' (Beattie 1991: 185). The collective focus of intervention emphasises the development of social relations and the articulation and sharing of experiences, problems and discontents. The aim is to engender a culture of collaboration and activism; mobilisation and emancipation of disempowered people as the social environment, rather than individual characteristics, is seen as the key determinant of health. The nurse as empowerment facilitator from a community/collective-action perspective also fits conceptually with the notion of co-production referred to by Cahn (1997) that includes the building of social infrastructures for self-help and of civic involvement for social health gain.

While Labonte (1993) contends that both are central to the 'new' public health, community-based work is not necessarily community development as defined above. It may also not be concerned with social capital, capacity building or participation. Some years prior to Labonte (1993), Beattie (1986) drew a similar conclusion and outlined four models of community practice that might be undertaken in the name of community development. In brief, and translated into health and social care, community outreach is a top-down method where external forces, for example, public health nurses, seek to determine the agenda of community health issues, push an official viewpoint or secure individual compliance on a health topic or in relation to health policies. It is akin to Arnstein's (1969) manipulation and therapy and token community participation and fits with the nurse as behaviour change agent for nurses with a community and public health brief. Community co-ordination is similarly top-down but with a collective focus and would involve public health nurses in integrating, co-ordinating and helping to ensure that health services, based on a professional community health needs assessment, are available and accessible to community members in need.

In line with the nurse as empowerment facilitator and his later personal counselling for health (Beattie 1991) and biographical health model (Beattie 1993), Beattie's (1986) diagram depicts community empowerment as a non-directive bottom-up but individually focused model of practice. It is to do with how members of a community interrelate, mutually assist each other and enhance social relations via involvement in local groups. However, these groups do not challenge local power structures or institutions that reinforce powerlessness (Beattie 1986) but may help individual group members develop personal skills to effect change in their personal life within a professional, health agency or institutional agenda. Finally, community action is a form of community mobilisation that fits more with community development as defined above by Labonte (1993), the Royal College of Nursing (2002) and Gilchrist (2007).

Thus, an understanding of the theory, models and techniques of community and psychosocial processes and ways to develop social capital may be used by public health nurses as a means to achieve pre-determined behavioural outcomes and a medical-model agenda. In other words, practice may be labelled community empowerment or community development but may be more about community outreach:

> Support from friends, family and health professionals can enhance physical health by encouraging health-promotion behaviour and discouraging poor health-related behaviours, such as over-eating. Conversely, lack of positive support – especially where there is negative pressure from other members of the social network – can lead to over-indulgence in risky behaviours, such as smoking, or undermine the individual's attempts to practise health-promoting behaviours, such as taking up exercise.
>
> (Cooper et al. 1999: 3)

Further to this, Muntainer et al. (2000) contend that social capital is a feature of the socio-political 'third way' of minimal government. When applied to public health it represents little more than an idealistic and romantic way to address social issues and has a questionable evidence-base for health gain. Its use of common-sense social psychology-approaches to engender better community relations in apparent conflict-free harmonious environments diverts attention away from structural problems such as socio-economic inequalities and the need for better welfare provision or the creation of jobs, etc.

Dinham (2005) observes that where there is success it tends to be at the level of personal development rather than community development, and doubts about the health outcomes of the latter approach (Dixon and Sindall 1994) and social capital have been noted (Gibson 2007). David et al. (1998) and Dinham (2005) also contend that it is wrong to assume that members of a community have the same aspirations or are indeed connected (Laverack 2005), while Muntainer et al. (2000) question whether strong social connectedness is always a good thing, for example, when operating among the criminal fraternity? In addition, Morrow (1999) questions whether it is feasible to simply take concepts from one cultural setting with different views on and structures for welfare provision, citizenship, community participation and local government such as the US and try to apply them in the UK?

Finally, the paradox is that although community development and social capital, etc., are being championed by the 'new' public health movement and health and social policy they may be out of step with contemporary cultural changes and the socio-political value system. Cooper *et al.* (1999) advance that the most widely used indicator of social capital is civic participation. Putnam (2000) points to a fall in civic participation and thus social capital since the Second World War in the US. He advances a number of reasons for this, including a preoccupation with personal goals and material acquisition, the decline of the traditional family and greater social mobility. Technology (for example, television and the internet) and the absence of major social movements such as flower power or world events such as VE (Victory in Europe) or VJ Day (Victory in Japan) around which people can unite have also played a part.

CONCLUSION

This chapter has considered the nature, purpose, methodologies and intended health gain of the process-orientated and radical-humanist nurse as empowerment facilitator from a collective-action perspective. It has undertaken a brief concept analysis of community, community empowerment and the social-action processes and key ways of working of community consultation, involvement, participation and collaboration and how they fit with community development. As can be seen from the preceding discussion, community empowerment, community development, social capital and capacity building can be used to describe various aspects of community practice, are not all-or-nothing concepts, can be enabled at different levels and reflect professional or lay agendas. However, in also focusing on ways to devolve control over health and health-related decision-making to communities the chapter has also outlined pragmatic enabling strategies for collective empowerment consistent with these concepts. This is in line with the developing 'new' public health agenda and evolving practice of public health nurses and those with a community remit.

LEARNING TRIGGERS

Having read Chapter 8, complete the learning triggers below to reinforce your understanding of the concepts that have been discussed:

- Define community and community empowerment.
- Summarise the key features of the community-action perspective of the nurse as empowerment facilitator model of health promotion.
- List examples of the aims, processes, impact and evaluation criteria and outcomes of intervention.
- Describe community consultation, involvement, participation and collaboration and differentiate between them.
- Define community development with reference to community development principles.
- Describe capacity-building and social capital.
- Summarise the pragmatic community-empowerment strategies for nurses.
- Summarise the socio-political and ideological foundations of the community-action perspective the nurse as empowerment facilitator model of health promotion.

THE NURSE AS STRATEGIC PRACTITIONER

INTRODUCTION

The focus of this chapter is the 'meso' (Tones and Tilford 2001: 9) patient population perspective of the nurse as strategic practitioner. As can be seen in Figure 5.1, it is a top-down, expert-directed form of intervention. Although mirroring the high nurse control of the nurse as behaviour change agent (Chapter 6), the nurse as strategic practitioner is not about individual patient-focused nurse–patient interaction on health-related behaviours or simply disease prevention. It is also not concerned with individual patient-focused nurse intervention to enhance personal control, autonomy or self-esteem or with empowering communities. The modus operandi of this model of health promotion is strategic, organisational and policy-based and thus focused on indirect intervention for health gain with associated socio-political values.

As was noted in Chapter 5, the concept of the nurse as strategic practitioner derives from one participant advancing this term when asked in Piper's (2004) interpretive inquiry testing the relationship between health promotion theory and nursing practice, how they would encapsulate the practice that they were describing. They were referring to their clinical setting collecting and interpreting data on presenting health care problems to identify and monitor patterns of mortality and morbidity and predisposing factors, causes and contexts. This evidence and other data were then fed back to appropriate sources, such as health agencies, local employers, local government or child-protection workers to highlight risk and influence change to help prevent further episodes.

However, although the nurse as strategic practitioner involves health surveillance and working at a multidisciplinary and multi-agency level and with industry for organisational, policy and operational change, strategic practice also translates into an intra-hospital internal operational and departmental agenda. It is then a settings approach that can work at different levels. From a nursing perspective it fits with the concept of Health Promoting Hospitals in general and Rushmere's (2000: 19) 'customer care' and Groene's (2006: 43, 38) 'patient information' and 'patient assessment' quality standards in particular.

Thus, in view of the fact that globally most nurses are employed in hospitals (Whitehead 2005d), this chapter will focus on the above and the related indicators and practical (i.e. not ideological/theoretical) examples of health promotion. It will include the aims, processes, impact and evaluatory criteria and outcomes to help illustrate this way of working in relation to nursing practice. As a model of practice it is worth noting that the settings approach can equally well be translated into other nursing milieus. Examples include schools, prisons, workplaces and communities (Hancock 1999; Tones and Green 2004) although they are likely to require different strategies for and modes of intervention (Dooris 2004).

LEARNING OUTCOMES

By reading this chapter, and completing the learning triggers at the end, the reader should have a better understanding of:

- the nurse as strategic practitioner model of health promotion;
- the aims, processes, impact and evaluation criteria and outcomes of intervention;
- health promotion from a strategic, policy, organisational and quality perspective;
- the concept of the Health Promoting Hospital in general and customer care, patient information and patient assessment in particular;
- the contribution that nurses can make to the above and to the concept of the Health Promoting Hospital at departmental level;
- the relationship between the nurse as strategic practitioner and empowerment;
- the socio-political and ideological foundations of the nurse as strategic practitioner and the associated barriers to developing a Health Promoting Hospital.

It is difficult to argue with Hancock's (1999: viii) contention that:

> it seems self-evident that a hospital should be a healing environ-
> ment, a healthy place to work, should not harm the health of the
> environment and should contribute to and be a source of health
> in the community.

However, historically health promotion was a marginal and fragmented
issue in hospitals (WHO 1991a, 1997b; Tones and Tilford 2001). The
health promotion conceptual shift beyond individuals (Whitelaw *et
al.* 2001; Dooris 2005) to populations, broader socio-political issues,
structural factors and the community in the physical and geographical
sense has helped change this. Hospitals are increasingly recognised
as an important, productive, trustworthy and credible place for health
promotion (WHO 1991a, 1997b; Naidoo and Wills 2000; Johnson
2000; Johnson and Baum 2001; Dooris and Hunter 2007).

Health Promoting Hospitals focus on populations (Dooris 2005)
and context in the form of institutional settings where individuals are
seen as relatively powerless and the power for change for health-gain
rests with organisations (Whitelaw *et al.* 2001). In acknowledging
that health is determined by organisational, environmental and
individual factors the Health Promoting Hospital philosophy reflects
ecological health promotion (Dooris 2005) and a shift in health
promotion towards a public health agenda. Pressure is growing for
all parts of health services and all health care professionals to address
wider health determinants and refocus to promote health both within
and without the physical boundaries of the hospital (Whitehead
2004b).

For Hancock (1999), health promotion as defined by the *Ottawa
Charter* (see Chapter 1) is concerned with both individual 'risk
factors' and social determinants of health. This translates into a
combination of:

- biomedical health promotion that aims to screen and treat
  individuals with 'risk factors' (for example, raised blood pressure);
- psychology-based health promotion for health-related behaviour
  change (for example, the nurse as behaviour change agent, see
  Chapter 6);
- socio-political and environmentally focused health promotion,
  which forms the foundation for the settings approach.

189

At one level, hospitals provide the opportunity for nurses to blend health promotion with other aspects of practice and work with patients more focused on health and illness and potentially more likely to be receptive to secondary-prevention input (Naidoo and Wills 2000; see Chapter 1 herein for definition of secondary prevention). They enable access to a significant proportion of the population (Kickham and Rushmere 1998; Wright *et al.* 2002; Dooris and Hunter 2007) and hence enable health promotion intervention not just for patients but also for relatives, visitors and the community. The Health Promoting Hospitals model of practice also endeavours to put health promotion more explicitly on the agenda by embedding it in the culture of all health care professionals (WHO 1991a, 1997b; Rushmere 2000).

At another level, and in line with Hancock (1999), it is important to stress that the concept of the Health Promoting Hospital takes health promotion beyond the narrow, traditional and medical model practice of the nurse as behaviour change agent (Chapter 6) and the health educating hospital (Whitehead 2004b). It is more than simply adding health promotion to a hospital's range of existing activities within established structures and value system (Johnson 2000) or having a few ad hoc (Kickham and Rushmere 1998) or unrelated (Whitehead 2004b) health promotion projects.

Health Promoting Hospitals is a WHO (1991a, 1997b) initiative that aims to further develop hospitals as health promotion settings beyond the above. The WHO *Budapest Declaration* (1991a) and the *Vienna Recommendations* (1997) suggest a more holistic vision of health. They encourage a shift in operational and decision-making philosophy beyond disease management and curative and care services. The intention is that hospitals should look for ways to contribute to disease prevention; an improvement in population health; and focus on process as well as clinical outcomes, but not at the expense of their traditional role.

Health Promoting Hospitals then go beyond simply providing lifestyle-related secondary health promotion following treatment and integrate clinical, educational, behavioural and organisational aspects of health care (Groene 2006). To be a Health Promoting Hospital means having health promotion and disease prevention as a core organisational value. The concept also transcends and cannot be delegated to any one staff group but is the responsibility of all health care professionals (Groene 2006).

Health Promoting Hospitals systematically integrate the theory, values and standards of health promotion into the corporate identity, strategic and organisational structure, culture and routine of the hospital and into the planning, development and delivery of services. This may result in the introduction of new, enhanced or re-engineered services to achieve health gain, efficient and cost-effective use of resources and, ideally, the development of a learning organisation culture (WHO 1997b).

ORGANISATIONAL DEVELOPMENT

For Dooris and Hunter (2007), hospitals are complex institutions influenced by their environment, stakeholders and by management and service delivery processes and systems. They contend that the culture of the medical model and the referent power of the medical profession, both in relation to other health care professionals and the public, together with managers lacking leadership skills are barriers to change. This may be compounded by bringing together diverse activities and groups under one banner ostensibly creating a consensus, when in reality, division (Whitelaw *et al.* 2001), a strict hierarchy and factional interests (Johnson 2000) exist.

Thus, to integrate health promotion theory, values and standards into the corporate identity, strategic and organisational structure, culture and routine of the hospital transformational managers are needed together with a systematic and informed process. To achieve the latter, the WHO (1997b) recommends the adoption of organisational development and project management methods and techniques.

Although the former is a contested concept it is summarised by Dooris and Hunter (2007) as the application of behavioural psychology for managing whole-organisational, group or individual transformation to improve performance and effectiveness. Dooris and Hunter (2007: 111) advance the four dimensions of 'environment and context, cultural change, skills development' and the 'structural development of systems and processes' to frame the settings approach to health promotion. This provides a structure to help facilitate organisational development for Health Promoting Hospitals.

Within this framework Dooris and Hunter (2007) give practical examples of indicators of the development of a health promotion infrastructure. These include job descriptions having health promotion written into them, health promotion being embedded in core business policy, health impact assessment and audit, and a contemporary cultural outlook and policies on employment practices such as flexible working and job sharing. Fielding and Woan (1998) echo this last indicator and highlight the inflexibility of shift patterns and rotas for nurses and suggest that turning hospitals into health promotion settings includes addressing these issues.

191

TYPES OF HEALTH PROMOTING SETTINGS

Dooris and Hunter (2007) and Whitelaw *et al.* (2001) note the impact on health promotion of the nature of the setting and how this varies between institutions inevitably determining the tone of the modus operandi of a Health Promoting Hospital. For example, as Whitelaw *et al.* (2001) point out, a health promotion setting with a top-down, authoritarian and centralised management structure and culture will be very different to one that is open and decentralised. Similarly, a setting that seeks to promote health within existing activities, skills and professional roles with pragmatic, short-term goals will deliver very different processes and outcomes to one that develops and nurtures flexible roles, a broader skill-base and more ambitious, longer term objectives.

As a result, the concept of the Health Promoting Hospital can be interpreted in various ways and its meaning contested (Johnson and Baum 2001). With differing modus operandi reflecting different philosophies and ways of working Whitelaw *et al.* (2001: 346) provide a most helpful break down of five models of health promoting settings that reflect variations in practice as summarised below:

- a 'passive' model where health promotion has an individual action perspective and the setting is simply a mode of access to, for example, patients, for the nurse as behaviour change agent-type (Chapter 6) interventions and outcomes;
- an 'active' model where the setting, while still pursuing an individual action perspective, provides resources and policy support to facilitate health promotion intervention and outcomes;
- a 'vehicle' model where the emphasis is on the setting and health promotion as a vehicle for policy and structural change;
- an 'organic' model that focuses on the setting as the cause of problems and individual action as providing the solutions;
- a 'comprehensive/structural' model where the setting is both the problem but also provides the means for solutions via policy and organisational change.

HEALTH PROMOTING HOSPITALS NETWORK

The WHO (1997b) recommend that Health Promoting Hospitals learn different ways of problem solving from the experience of peer organisations embarking on similar changes or from those that have progressed further along this path. Membership of regional, national and international organisations such as the WHO Health Promoting Hospitals European Network is encouraged. The WHO require that member hospitals:

- sign up to the principles and strategies of the *Vienna Recommendations;*
- are members of regional and national networks where these are established;
- comply with the regional, national and international rules and regulations of the members of the network and the WHO;
- utilise the WHO *Standards for Health Promotion in Hospitals* toolkit (WHO 2004) for self-assessment and the identification of priorities for intervention (Dooris and Hunter 2007).

In addition, member hospitals have to develop a minimum of five health promotion five-year projects and collaborate with an academic or research institution for independent monitoring and evaluation of the projects (Naidoo and Wills 2000). Examples of health topic areas for intervention include environmentally responsible energy and waste management and product purchasing (WHO 1997b; Dooris and Hunter 2007), hospital hygiene, smoking, alcohol and diet and nutrition (Fielding and Woan 1998), exercise and physical fitness and occupational health (Health Education Authority 1993; Wright *et al.* 2002).

HEALTH PROMOTING HOSPITALS AND QUALITY

The Health Promoting Hospital aims to improve patient satisfaction and the effectiveness, efficiency, equity and thus quality of health care (WHO 1997b; Rushmere 2000). A framework for the latter, and thus for health promotion in hospital, can be achieved by rationalising quality to the standards in Box 9.1.

Standards and indicators of health promotion should be built into and seen as adding value to other quality management processes (Groene 2006; Dooris and Hunter 2007) and should be incorporated into existing service provision (Naidoo and Wills 2000). The WHO (1991a, 1997b) philosophy of Health Promoting Hospitals requires a healthy organisational culture and structure that rejects orthodox, hierarchical management in favour of inclusive ways of working and decision-making that is transparent (Dooris and Hunter 2007). As well as management, hospital staff (including staff representatives such as trade unions) and patient/public representatives should play an active part in the latter (WHO 1991a, 1997b; Dooris and Hunter 2007).

The *Vienna Recommendations* (WHO 1997b) acknowledge that working in a hospital exposes staff to hazardous chemicals, infection and stress and are equally concerned to improve the health, working conditions and job satisfaction of staff. Thus, and in relation to the above, for the WHO, among other things the Health Promoting Hospital is concerned with:

- the ambience created by the physical and working environment of the hospital for patients, staff and visitors; risk reduction; the quality of catering and hotel services; and how these factors can assist the healing process, reduce staff sickness, stress and burnout and improve recruitment and retention;
- promoting active patient participation and empowerment, patients' rights, human dignity, equity, recognition of different value sets and cultural needs, and professional ethics;
- the provision and quality of information, communication styles and educational programmes and skills training for patients, staff and relatives;
- inter-professional co-operation and communication, collaboration and building alliances with the community at two levels. First, with health and social care services, support groups and organisations to enhance the range of support given to patients and their relatives. Second, with local health promotion programmes including the Healthy Cities Network;
- hospitals developing a public health role including generating an epidemiological data base concerned with disease and injury prevention and communicating the findings to public policy makers and community services.

HEALTH PROMOTING HOSPITALS AND NURSING PRACTICE

In Whitehead's (2005d) view, although nursing has been championed as the professional group to lead health promotion within health services the profession has failed to rise to this challenge both in general and in relation to Health Promoting Hospitals in particular. He contends that as the largest professional group, nursing is in a good position to facilitate health promotion and engage with the wider health promotion agenda and should use the Health Promoting Hospitals concept as an opportunity to broaden practice beyond that of the nurse as behaviour change agent. However, Whitehead (2005d) does acknowledge that the complex management structure of a hospital setting may exclude nurses from involvement in more strategic health promotion. Robinson and Hill (1999) contend that this is impeded by a combination of factors. These include poor health promotion knowledge and skills in nursing, a lack of nursing time, inadequate nursing management and multidisciplinary working and pathological hospital environments. Johnson (2000) echoes the sentiment pertaining to inadequate training but extends this to all health care professionals.

The implications of this are that first, nurses must become more political, advocacy-focused and prepared to challenge institutional processes when trying to push for change within the categories referred to earlier. Second, those nurses in management positions must facilitate the development of the health promotion skills of nurses, multidisciplinary practice and ways to improve the working environment of health care professionals (Robinson and Hill 1999).

In general, health promotion policy and practice development in nursing ranges from healthy eating to discharge planning (Latter 2001). Lask (1987) suggests targeting key groups such as pensioners, mothers and self-help groups and key processes in nursing settings such as improving the structure and organisation of hospital admissions. Nurses can strive to organise practice to reflect holistic health needs and provide continuity of care (Fielding and Woan 1998). Consideration can also be given to the organisation of outpatient clinics in relation to the time allowed for consultation, the time between these, the physical environment, privacy and the workload of health care professionals (Department of Health 2004c).

Nurses can play an instrumental part in hospitals role-modelling good practice via outreach projects on heart disease and diabetes (Naidoo and Wills 2000). In addition, a network of health promotion link nurses could be developed across the hospital to catalyse and monitor health promotion activity in their clinical settings. Health promotion could be a part of the performance appraisal and review of the link nurses who should be given the opportunity to attend health promotion courses to facilitate this role.

More specifically, while seeking to contribute to the Health Promoting Hospital general agenda focusing on management, workplace, facilities, environment, community involvement and partnership (Rushmere 2000) issues, customer care (Rushmere 2000), patient information and patient assessment (Groene 2006) have a more obvious and direct relevance for the nurse as strategic practitioner.

Rushmere (2000) defines the customer as the patient and the carer. The contention of this chapter is that nursing, because of the one-to-one interpersonal nature of practice, is the ideal professional group to provide a strategic lead on the implementation and audit of indicators of effective practice within the customer care (Rushmere 2000), patient information and patient assessment (Groene 2006) standards. This type of health promotion would be consistent with the UK Department of Health (2006b) benchmark for promoting health concerned with access to information and the UK NHS Executive. As far back as 1994 the latter were citing literature extolling the benefits that could be delivered, such as a reduction in pre-operative anxiety, more rapid post-surgery recovery and a greater uptake of prescribed medication (NHS Management Executive 1994).

The customer care of Rushmere (2000) overlaps with Groene's (2006) patient information standard in including the provision of quality information. To help illustrate how these fit with the nurse as strategic practitioner the aim, processes, impact and thus evaluatory criteria (see Chapter 5) to help establish an evidence-base (Dooris and Hunter 2007) and outcomes of this facet of the model are summarised in Table 9.1.

Groene's (2006: 43) patient information standard states that:

> The organisation provides patients with information on significant factors concerning their disease or health condition and health promotion interventions are established in all patient pathways.

The similarly expressed objectives are concerned to keep the patient informed, to empower and work in partnership with them and integrate health promotion into all aspects of patient care. The role of the nurse as strategic practitioner is not to deliver patient information in the way that the nurse as behaviour change agent does but to put structures in place to facilitate this and monitor practice. This can be achieved by using Groene's (2006: 45) measurable and auditable indicators of the standard such as:

Table 9.1 The nurse as strategic practitioner

Aims	Processes	Impact and evaluation indicators	Outcomes and evaluation indicators
Quality patient information as part of customer care (Rushmere 2000, Groene 2006)	Hospital/department policy development for integrated patient information	Provision of and access to integrated patient information	Informed patient
		Patient information conforms to quality	Patient satisfaction
Health promoting clinical setting	Development of patient information quality standards	standards and is: • speciality specific; • culturally sensitive; • available in different languages; • regularly reviewed and updated (Rushmere 2000)	Reduced: mortality; morbidity; injury; disability; complications; (Piper 2007b); complaints
	Organisational and policy development and implementation and service management	Right staff, right place, right time, right skill mix	
		Evidence-based practice including the use of national/international guidelines and protocols	
		Multidisciplinary team working and training	

- percentage of patients educated about specific actions in self-management of their condition;
- per cent of patients educated about risk factor modification and disease treatment options in the management of their condition.

Groene (2006) advances a number of concomitant substandards that are also in effect auditable indicators of practice that fit well with a nursing agenda and which include ensuring that:

- health promotion intervention was documented in the patient's notes, i.e. what information was given to the patient and its expected impact;
- the level of patient satisfaction with the health promotion intervention was documented in the patient's notes;
- the hospital population have access to information on health determinants;
- patients, relatives and carers have access to information on support groups, etc.

Tones and Tilford (2001) share the view that health promotion should be documented with other aspects of health care following intervention, but add that as well as being retrospective it should be prospective with health promotion needs being identified in the care plan. All of this requires nurses to have a positive attitude to this aspect of practice and acknowledge the information needs of their patients, which might include, for example, information on disease aetiology, diagnosis and prognosis, the inpatient experience, rehabilitation and sources of support. However, to move beyond individual practitioner variations in commitment and performance to achieve strategic success necessitates organisational arrangements to facilitate intervention. It requires the development of policy specifying patient information as a key aspect of practice and detailing how this should be achieved and appropriate staff training (Tones and Tilford 2001).

Groene's (2006) patient assessment standard, applied to nursing, would focus on ensuring that nurses work in partnership with patients to assess health promotion needs with the objective of supporting treatment, improving outcomes and promoting their general health and well-being. There are three key indicators that measure the percentage of patients that have been assessed for generic and disease-specific risk factors and gauge the level of patient satisfaction with the assessment process.

As with patient information, Groene (2006) advances a number of patient assessment substandards that equate with auditable indicators of practice and that similarly fit well with a nursing agenda. They include ensuring the deployment of general guidelines for assessing and reassessing health promotion needs in relation, for example, to smoking, alcohol and diet, disease-specific guidelines for asthma, diabetes, chronic obstructive pulmonary disease, surgery, etc., and discharge from hospital. These, together with evidence of sensitivity to socio-cultural experiences (Groene 2006) and the health promotion needs assessment, must be documented in the patient's notes.

For Rushmere (2000), customer care also includes ensuring that mechanisms (for example nurse training and clinical audit) are in place to ensure:

* shared decision-making;
* that the customer voice is heard and is influential both in individual health-related matters and in relation to service development;
* that customers know how to make a complaint and raise concerns about inadequate care or service provision;
* that customers are afforded the opportunity to choose whether or not they want to participate in medical research and medical student training;
* that lifestyle risk factors are discussed with patients at all stages of care.

Additional Health Promoting Hospital quality indicators within the nursing sphere of influence focus on making the inpatient experience as comfortable as possible. Examples include ensuring that patients have access to a telephone, TV, radio and loop system, flexible visiting times, refreshments available outside of mealtimes, facilities for special needs, interpretation services and guidance documentation on the needs of patients from different ethnic backgrounds (Rushmere 2000).

HEALTH PROMOTING HOSPITAL DEPARTMENT

Although it must be remembered that clinical-practice settings are but a small part of a hospital and the bigger picture, i.e. a whole organisation perspective, should not be forgotten, the ward or department is an important focus for health promotion by nurses (Whitehead 2005d). Fielding and Woan (1998) concur in referring to one hospital where nurses were the lead practitioners for health promotion at this level and Piper (2007b) applies this concept to emergency (A&E) nursing.

Piper's (2007b) examples are used here to illustrate the potential application of the nurse as strategic practitioner to departmental, i.e. indirect, health promotion practice consistent with the Health Promoting Hospitals ethos. He suggests that first, emergency nurses can address wider health issues outwith the department by lobbying national and local politicians through their professional organisations and specialist forums and align themselves with other pressure groups. This can be on issues such as poverty and welfare provision, car design, drinking and driving, health and safety laws governing the workplace and advertising bans on products deleterious to health.

Second, and with a specific departmental focus, Piper (2007b) suggests that the nurse as strategic practitioner can be applied from an organisational perspective to promote population health gain. Intervention could focus on quality, standards of practice and the management of emergency department resources such as skill mix and the deployment of senior staff to maximise health gain. The latter can be measured by, for example, trauma scoring.

In addition, clinical governance, education and training, collaborative care planning and evidence-based practice including the use of nationally recognised protocols such as those for advanced life support, asthma, etc., and appropriate directives from the UK National Service Frameworks contribute to enhanced clinical outcomes. The feasibility of service developments and their potential for health gain, such as the establishment of trauma teams, could also be explored (Piper 2007b). To illustrate this aspect of the nurse as strategic practitioner the aim, together with examples of the process, impact and thus evaluatory criteria and outcomes are summarised in Table 9.1. Action research methodology may also lend itself well to developing and evaluating health promotion activity of this nature (Whitehead 2004b).

STRATEGIC EMPOWERMENT

Although empowerment is essentially an individual or community-focused bottom-up process as discussed at length in Chapters 7 and 8 respectively, there are institutional and strategic interventions that can be undertaken by health service management and nurses that can help facilitate the process. The NHS Management Executive (1993), albeit from the annals of UK NHS policy development, restrict their pragmatic definition of patient empowerment to a shift in the balance of power towards service users and away from service providers. This laudable but limited definition, which omits to define the desired extent of the shift in the balance of power, has the seven key goals outlined in Box 9.2.

Whereas the second and fourth as practical processes involve ensuring access to interpreters and informal and formal patient advocates and champions, the third focuses on the patient's right to make decisions about what happens to them and is advanced as a fundamental right. Fair redress is about empowering patients to make complaints, although the process for enabling this is not clarified. Participation in planning seeks to canvass the views of patients and their representatives on service provision and service developments and involve these in standard setting, monitoring and evaluating the quality of service key goal.

With regard to the latter, Wilson (1999/2000) outlines how the patients' panel has been set up at one hospital. The patients' panel is a mechanism for canvassing the views of service users when planning, delivering and monitoring services, with the concept of partnership central to business planning and individual objectives. There is now a requirement for UK NHS Trusts (hospital and community service providers) to ensure this type of patient participation, to publish an annual prospectus and create a patients' forum to provide input into service management (Department of Health 2004c). The UK Department of Health (2004c) add that the way clinics and consultations are organised makes an important contribution to facilitating and inhibiting patient involvement.

BOX 9.2 THE SEVEN KEY PATIENT EMPOWERMENT GOALS OF THE NHS MANAGEMENT EXECUTIVE

The goals are concerned with:

1 maximising available information
2 equality of access
3 respect for personal autonomy
4 representation
5 participation in planning
6 quality of service
7 fair redress.

NHS Management Executive (1993)

There is a fair degree of conceptual fit between the nurse as strategic practitioner, Beattie's (1993) ecological model of health and his analysis of this in relation to the grid/group analysis of Douglas (1982) and its high grid/high group position. It represents a culture of control and environment management concerned with the health of a population rather than of individuals.

The ecological model of health and the associated legislative action for health (Beattie 1991) model of health promotion contend that social and environmental factors are major determinants of health status. The poor health experiences and higher accident rates of the lower occupational groups are ascribed to class differentials and concomitant socio-economic inequalities including the unequal distribution of income, wealth and capital (Townsend *et al.* 1988; Acheson 1998). Health promotion is concerned to improve the health of populations through health, social, economic, industrial, environmental and agricultural legislation. It includes the development of policies for risk management (Beattie 1993; Rushmere 2000), social and welfare provision and traditional public health interventions. Persuasive advertising can also be monitored and laws can be enacted to control the perceived harmful effects of products.

While the nurse as strategic practitioner is concerned with the above, i.e. macro social intervention on legislative, environmental and public health issues and a socio-political agenda, the emphasis is on 'meso' (Tones and Tilford 2001: 9) health promotion practice for population, i.e. hospital or department population health gain. However, it can fit conceptually with Beattie's (1991, 1993) analysis and models of health and health promotion if its socio-political centralist and bureaucratic ideology translates into strategic, policy and organisational interventions based on professionally assessed needs and associated aims, processes, impact and outcomes of practice.

Thus, the nurse as strategic practitioner is asymmetric with the practitioner maintaining a 'high social distance' (Beattie 1991: 187). Indeed the nature of some of the Health Promoting Hospitals quality initiatives in being management-focused and hierarchical may create rather than reduce barriers to organisational change and thus contradict the health promotion settings ethos (Whitehead 2004b) and undermine any efforts to empower (Johnson 2000). This is reinforced by a sharper focus on the medical model in terms of acute care at the expense of non-acute beds and making ever-greater efforts to make hospitals run with mechanistic efficiency (Robinson and Hill 1999).

The contradiction to the ideology underpinning Health Promoting Hospitals is fuelled by hospital routines, a crisis intervention culture, the disease focus of these settings and increasingly highly technical medical practice (Johnson 2000). These create an environment alien to the public and exacerbate further patient disempowerment (Johnson 2000) as a result of this medicalisation, individualisation and institutionalisation (Hancock 1999).

CONCLUSION

This chapter has discussed the nature, aim, processes, impact and evaluatory criteria and health outcomes of the nurse as strategic practitioner together with a brief socio-political critique. A general overview of the concept of the Health Promoting Hospital has been presented, which involves embedding the theory, values and quality standards of health promotion into hospital culture, strategy, policy and health care practice and into the planning and development of services. The Health Promoting Hospital way of working has also been translated into interventions at a departmental level. In addition, this chapter has advanced that nursing can take the health promotion lead in the areas of customer care, patient information and patient assessment.

203

LEARNING TRIGGERS

Having read Chapter 9, complete the learning triggers below to reinforce your understanding of the concepts that have been discussed:

- Summarise the key features of the nurse as strategic practitioner model of health promotion.
- List examples of the aims, processes, impact and evaluation criteria and outcomes of intervention.
- Define the concept of the Health Promoting Hospital and describe how intervention from a strategic, policy, organisational and quality perspective can promote health.
- Describe the customer care, patient information and patient assessment aspects of the Health Promoting Hospital and the contribution that nurses can make to these quality standards.
- Describe the contribution that nurses can make to the Health Promoting Hospital at a departmental level.
- Define strategic empowerment.
- Summarise the socio-political and ideological foundations of the nurse as strategic practitioner and the associated barriers to developing a Health Promoting Hospital.

CONCLUSION

The ideas for this book were initiated and have evolved against a health and professional policy backdrop increasingly emphasising the health promotion aspect of nursing practice. This has been accompanied by a shift in nurse education philosophy from a disease model to a health model. In addition, the nursing literature clearly demonstrates that health education and health promotion are an acknowledged part of the repertoire of nursing language and practice. Thus, the dialogue and concepts associated with these are not entirely foreign to nurses. In light of this, the book has set out first, to help clarify the meaning and enhance further our understanding of health promotion and related concepts. Second, to offer for consideration a research driven, robust, inclusive and integrated framework of models for contextualising, mapping and guiding 'real world', i.e. theoretically informed pragmatic nursing health promotion practice.

THEORETICAL TRANSFERABILITY, TRUSTWORTHINESS AND 'REAL WORLD' NURSING

It is acknowledged that theoretical analysis, theory development and research are never independent of interpretation. All are influenced by the author's background, values and ideological world view, and this book is no different in reflecting a personal interpretation and construction of reality. This being the case, it is incumbent on the reader to engage in a dialogue with and challenge the text, the analysis and assertions of the book in relation to their patient/client group, practice setting, clinical and/or professional focus and perspective. This will enable judgements to be made about the transferability of the health promotion framework and models to the reader's 'real world' of nursing.

The potential for transferability derives from trustworthiness. Trustworthiness is conferred when the reader is convinced by clear explanation, transparency of the socio-political/philosophical perspectives, the theoretical and research processes and the relevance of the findings. Trustworthiness and the degree of transferability, then, are a matter of reader interpretation and judgement and not of shared interpretation.

To facilitate trustworthiness and the potential for transferability, Chapter 1 defined the contested concepts of health, health education, health promotion and public health consistent with the general literature and health policy. It was important to start at this theoretical juncture to enable the reader to gain a clear understanding of the meaning given to these concepts in the book. It was also important because if nursing wants to influence policy and practice it must use mainstream terminology or it will not be heard by other disciplines, managers, policy makers or academic fields of enquiry. This argument applies equally to nurse education and for the same reasons.

Chapter 2 endeavoured to address the trustworthiness and transferability of the health promotion framework and models of the book by providing operational definitions of these concepts and associated terminology. It outlined levels of theorising and the relationship between theory and models to help avoid ambiguity and contextualise the theoretical debate. Chapter 2 also identified and applied the criteria that were used for internal theory testing to judge, compare and contrast the rigour, breadth and depth of health promotion frameworks.

This process illuminated how Beattie's (1991) framework of health promotion models came to be advanced. Essentially this was because of its potential to serve as a benchmark by which to measure others and as a foundation for developing and synthesising a tool for nursing practice as per the work of Piper and Brown (1998a) and Piper (2000, 2004, 2007a, 2007b). The socio-political and socio-cultural analysis and synthesis was assisted by the complementary frameworks and models of health (Beattie 1993) and cultural bias (Douglas 1982). Beattie's (1991) health promotion framework proved to have a number of strengths. It had both factor-isolating and factor-relating properties and stood up to the demands of internal theory testing to good effect. The internal structure of Beattie's (1991) framework and the relationship between its inherent models was described subsequently together with their mode and focus of intervention.

A critical review and evaluation of key, mainstream literature on competing health education/promotion frameworks was undertaken in Chapter 3 to test further and force a reconsideration of Beattie's (1991) work as the benchmark framework. For the same reasons, this process and format was repeated in Chapter 4 but specifically in relation to nursing. In addition, to help gain an understanding of the health promotion modus operandi of nurses and nursing, Chapter 4 reviewed studies undertaken on nursing and health education/promotion that highlighted predominantly traditional forms of practice.

From this it was concluded that although the conceptual devices competing with Beattie's (1991) work suggested ostensibly a broad range of health education and health promotion frameworks, they were for the most part variations on a theme. By comparison, most were descriptive, pragmatic and factor-isolating and limited in their breadth, depth and levels of theoretical analysis. In the main, they lacked reference to epistemological and methodological considerations, socio-political philosophy and socio-cultural theory and thus what their inherent models represent from an ideological perspective. These authors were not interested in advancing a comprehensive and detailed health promotion framework; their primary concern was with creating a backdrop for discussion or in outlining a preferred perspective or principles of practice. Although some authors were excused the criticisms above by drawing on an established framework of social theory, most were more tentative, none had the clarity, precision and potential for specific and detailed application of Beattie (1991) and few exposed the theoretical assumptions of their work with such rigour.

Building on the work of previous chapters and to facilitate further the potential for trustworthiness and transferability into 'real world' nursing, Chapter 5 provided a full explanation of the health promotion framework of the book, its inherent health promotion models and the relationship between them (Figure 5.1). It described how the framework was synthesised and derived from Beattie's (1991) work and frameworks for nursing explicitly based on this (Piper and Brown 1998a; Piper 2000, 2004, 2007a, 2007b), qualitative theory testing research (Piper 2004) and additional theorising.

Chapter 5 went on to translate into practice the methodologies, methods and outcomes of the models and thus a repertoire of approaches that can be operationalised by nurses in their various practice settings. These were subsequently developed further in Part 2 of the book in Chapters 6, 7, 8 and 9, focusing on practice.

207

In addition, Chapter 5 acknowledged that 'real world' nursing requires not only theory for practice but pragmatic strategies for evaluating intervention. To this end, health promotion models evaluation categories and criteria in general with emphasis on impact (intermediate outcomes) in particular were outlined.

Chapter 5 also described in brief and defined the qualitative methods of Piper's (2004) research testing the relationship between health promotion theory and nursing practice. The findings were, of course, limited by the purposive sampling of 32 participants, their age range, gender and ethnicity. The fieldwork took place in a particular era and, with the exception of one participant, with qualified general nurses working in the same acute hospital. The findings also reflect a particular time, setting and policy agenda and the views of a particular group of people and, in line with the concepts of trustworthiness and transferability in qualitative research, no claims of generalisability are made.

The idea was simply to give some insight into Piper's (2004) qualitative research processes that inductively generated a set of findings that were used to help develop and test the health promotion framework of the book. The central theme of the nurse as informer underpinned all aspects of practice of the complementary themes that formed the models of the framework (Figure 5.1) and thus the chapters of Part 2 (practice) of the book as follows:

- the nurse as behaviour change agent (Chapter 6);
- the nurse as empowerment facilitator (Chapters 7 and 8);
- the nurse as strategic practitioner (Chapter 9).

As was discussed in Chapter 5, the virtue of the framework for 'real world' nursing is that it highlights issues of power and control, contrasting socio-political and philosophical foundations and contradictory and shared agendas of the models of health promotion. For example, the nurse as behaviour change agent and the nurse as empowerment facilitator with an individual action perspective do invoke different aims, methods, impact and evaluatory criteria and outcomes and are polarised on the power continuum. However, to suggest that they are mutually exclusive and in complete opposition would represent only a superficial analysis and a premature conclusion. Similarly, although the former shares its position on the power continuum and top-down approach to practice with the nurse as strategic practitioner, it has a divergent population focus of intervention and yet may ultimately help achieve the intended impact and outcomes of the nurse as behaviour change agent.

ORIGINALITY

This book has sought to make a unique contribution to the development of nursing health promotion theory and knowledge in a number of ways: first, through internal theory testing via the application of intellectually sound criteria developed in other fields of academic endeavour to evaluate the strengths and limitations of frameworks of health promotion models; second, through drawing on the findings of Piper's (2004) interpretive study that tested and described the degree of fit between the themes from fieldwork data and existing health promotion frameworks, models and theory; third, via metatheoretical analysis of the socio-political philosophies and socio-cultural perspectives, theory derivation and synthesis, by which a health promotion framework has been advanced tentatively as a conceptual framework for classifying and contextualising nursing practice.

For nursing to develop a more holistic type of health promotion and embrace a repertoire of approaches, there is a need for theoretical frameworks that enable an understanding of the assumptions underpinning the focus, mode and model of intervention to inform and facilitate practice and practice development. This book has contributed to this process by the original use of existing frameworks of health promotion models as a basis for theory derivation and thus theory development in nursing.

In addition, and in line with Beattie's (1991) prediction for all health and social care professions, in its derived theory state the framework as a classification scheme identifies the main terms of reference for self-scrutiny by nurses and nursing. If this assertion is taken to its logical conclusion the revised framework, with appropriately modified terminology to reflect the discipline under scrutiny, could also make an original contribution to the discourse of other health and social care professions in the early stages of developing theoretical frameworks for practice.

THE WAY FORWARD: IMPLICATIONS FOR PRACTICE, FURTHER RESEARCH AND EDUCATION

The nursing literature identifies health promotion as an important element of practice and there are a plethora of descriptive, factor-isolating frameworks available for use. However, those that are theory tested, take account of their theoretical foundations and derivations in relation to existing structures, are based on inductive processes and explicitly contextualise their inherent models in relation to socio-political theory, practitioner–patient/client locus of control and individual/population perspectives, are notable by their absence.

Hence, this book has endeavoured to redress this situation and advance a research-driven health promotion framework based on these processes as a template that can be used to help nurses identify, chart and plan clinically focused interventions and strategic, organisational and patient-led processes. Nevertheless, it is acknowledged, in line with the thoughts of Silva and Rothbart (1984), that the derived health promotion framework advanced herein represents no more than a stage in the partial development of theory in nursing and is not the final contribution to this particular debate. It is not a fully tested or saturated factor-relating theory and thus not a set of fixed and ever-lasting truths. It will require additional research with nurses in a multitude of practice settings and with all levels of the nursing hierarchy to test the theory/practice relationship and the durability, trustworthiness and thus potential transferability of the derived framework.

For example, similar research in a different acute hospital would help test further this degree of fit, as would a study undertaken with participants in a completely different setting where particular aspects of the findings could be subjected to scrutiny. An obvious example would be fieldwork with health visitors and school nurses in the community, exploring how they are developing the public health role required of them by UK health policy to test the framework in general and the nurse as empowerment facilitator from a community action perspective in particular.

The health promotion framework of this book also has implications for the 'real world' of teaching nurses and thus the practice of nurse educators. Nurses engage in a repertoire of health promotion interventions and these need to be disseminated for consideration and peer review by nurses so that they can consider the potential for transferability, change and development in their own practice. This process can be complemented by the use of the health promotion framework of the book (Chapter 5, Figure 5.1) in two ways. First, by elucidating the distinctions and overlap between the models identified and their discrete positions in relation to locus of control and focus of intervention. Second, by its use as a framework to structure an educational encounter in the form of Ausubel's 'advance organiser' introduced prior to the introduction of teaching material to anchor the content (Quinn 1995). Finally, and at the risk of repetition, to help nurses understand and contribute to the general health promotion debate, nurse education needs to use terminology compatible with that of other disciplines, the general literature and health policy (Piper 2008).

REFERENCES

Abelin, T. (1987) 'Approaches to health promotion and disease prevention', in Abelin, T., Brzezinski, Z.J. and Carstairs, V.D.L. (eds) *Measurement in Health Promotion and Health Protection.* Copenhagen: WHO Regional Publications, European Series. No. 22.

Abercrombie, N., Hill, S. and Turner, B.S. (1988) *Dictionary of Sociology*, London: Penguin.

Acheson, D. (1988) *Public Health in England: The report of the Committee of Inquiry into the future developments of the public health function*, London: HMSO.

Acheson, D. (1998) *Independent Inquiry into Inequalities in Health Report*, London: Stationery Office.

Adam, E. (1985) 'Toward more clarity in terminology: frameworks, theories and models.' *Journal of Nursing Education*, 24 (4): 151–5.

Adams, L. and Pintus, S. (1994) 'A challenge to prevailing theory and practice.' *Critical Public Health*, 5 (2): 17–29.

Allender, J.A. and Spradley, B.W. (2005) *Community Health Nursing: promoting the public's health* (6th edn), Philadelphia, PA: Lippincott Williams.

American Nurses Association (2007) *Health of the Public*. http://nursingworld. org/MainMenuCategories/HealthcareandPolicyIssues/HoP.aspx (accessed 18 October 2007).

Anderson, R. (1983) *Health Promotion: an overview*. Unit technical paper prepared for the Regional Office for Europe of the WHO, Copenhagen, Denmark.

Anderson, R. (1984) 'Health promotion: an overview', in Baric, L. (ed.) *European Monographs in Health Education Research*. Scottish Health Education Group pamphlet.

Arnstein, S.R. (1969) 'A ladder of citizen participation.' *AIP Journal*, July: 216–24.

Baggott, R. (2000) *Public Health: policy and politics*, Basingstoke: Palgrave Macmillan.

Baggott, R. (2004) *Health and Health Care in Britain*, Basingstoke: Palgrave Macmillan.

Ballard, K. and Elston, A. (2005) 'Medicalisation: a multi-dimensional concept.' *Social Theory and Health*, 3: 228–41.

Baraitser, P., Fettiplace, R., Dolan, F., Massil, H. and Cowley, S. (2002) 'Quality, mainstream services with proactive and targeted outreach: a model of contraceptive service provision for young people.' *The Journal of Family Planning and Reproductive Health Care*, 29 (2): 90–3.

Baric, L. (1982) 'A new ecological perspective emerging for health education.' *The Journal of the Institute of Health Education*, 20 (4): 5–21.

Baric, L. (1985) 'The meaning of words: health promotion.' *The Journal of the Institute of Health Education*, 23 (1): 10–16.

Beattie, A. (1986) 'Community development for health: from practice to theory?' *Radical Health Promotion*, Summer/Autumn (4): 12–18.

Beattie, A. (1991) 'Knowledge and control in health promotion: a test case for social policy and social theory', in Gabe, J., Calnan, M. and Bury, M. (eds) *The Sociology of the Health Service*, London: Routledge.

Beattie, A. (1993) 'The changing boundaries of health,' in Beattie, A., Gott, M. Jones, L. and Sidell, M. (eds) *Health and Wellbeing*, Milton Keynes: OU Press.

Benner, P. (1983) 'Uncovering the knowledge embedded in clinical practice image.' *The Journal of Nursing Scholarship*, Spring, XV (2): 36–41.

Benner, P. (1984) *From Novice to Expert: excellence and power in clinical nursing practice*, Menlo Park, CA: Addison-Wesley.

Benner, P. and Wrubel, J. (1989) *The Primacy of Caring: stress and coping in health and illness*, Menlo Park, CA: Addison-Wesley.

Benson, A. and Latter, S. (1998) 'Implementing health promoting nursing: the integration of interpersonal skills and health promotion.' *Journal of Advanced Nursing*, 27: 100–7.

Berg, G.V. and Sarvimäki, A. (2003) 'A holistic-existential approach to health promotion.' *Scandinavian Journal of Caring Sciences*, 17: 384–91.

Berland, A., Whyte, N.B. and Maxwell, L. (1995) 'Hospital nurses and health promotion.' *Canadian Journal of Nursing Research*, 27 (4): 13–31.

Betz, C.L. (2006) 'Surgical preoperative preparation for children: the need for more evidence from nurse scientists.' *Journal of Pediatric Nursing*, 21 (6): 397–9.

Bircher, A.U. (1975) 'On the development and classification of diagnosis.' *Nursing Forum*, XIV (1): 10–29.

Blackburn, C. (1991) *Poverty and Health: working with families*, Milton Keynes: OU Press.

Breuera, E., Sweeney, C., Calder, K., Palmer, L. and Benisch-Tolley, S. (2001) 'Patient preferences versus physician perceptions of treatment decisions in cancer care.' *Journal of Clinical Oncology*, 19 (11): 2883–5.

Brown, E.R. and Margo, G.E. (1978) 'Health education: can the reformers be reformed?' *International Journal of Health Services*, 8 (1): 3–26.

Brown, P.A. and Piper, S.M. (1997) 'Nursing and the health of the nation: schism or symbiosis?.' *Journal of Advanced Nursing*, 25: 297–301.

Brubaker, B.H. (1983) 'Health promotion: a linguistic analysis.' *Advances in Nursing Science*, 5: 1–14.

Bunton, R. and Macdonald, G. (1992) *Health Promotion: disciplines and diversity*, London: Routledge.

Bunton, R. and Macdonald, G. (2002) *Health Promotion: disciplines and diversity* (2nd edn), London: Routledge.

Burke, L.M. and Smith, P. (2000) 'Developing an audit tool for health promotion learning opportunities in clinical placements.' *Nurse Education Today*, 20: 475–84.

Burkitt, A. (1983) 'Health education', in Clark, J. and Henderson, J. (eds) *Community Health*, London: Churchill Livingstone.

Burrell, G. and Morgan, G. (1979) *Sociological Paradigms and Organisational Analysis*, London: Heinemann.

Byrt, R. and Dooher, J. (2002) 'Empowerment and participation: definitions, meanings and models', in Dooher, J. and Byrt, R. (eds) *Empowerment and Participation: power, influence and control in contemporary health care. Volume One.* Trowbridge: Quay Books.

Cahill, J. (1996) 'Patient participation: a concept analysis.' *Journal of Advanced Nursing*, 24: 561–71.

Cahn, E.S. (1997) 'The co-production imperative.' *Social Policy*, 27 (3): 62–7.

Campbell, T. (1981) *Seven Theories of Human Society*, Oxford: Clarendon Press.

Campbell, T.A., Auerbach, S.M. and Kiesler, D.J. (2007) 'Relationship of interpersonal behaviours and health-related control appraisals to patient satisfaction and compliance in a university health centre.' *Journal of American College Health*, 55 (6): 333–40.

Caplan, R. (1993) 'The importance of social theory for health promotion: from description to reflexivity.' *Health Promotion International*, 8 (2): 147–57.

Caplan, R. and Holland, R. (1990) 'Rethinking health education theory.' *Health Education Journal*, 49 (1): 10–12.

Caraher, M. (1994a) 'Health promotion: time for an audit.' *Nursing Standard*, 8 (20): 32–5.

Caraher, M. (1994b) 'A sociological approach to health promotion for nurses in an institutional setting.' *Journal of Advanced Nursing*, 20: 544–51.

Caraher, M. (1994c) 'Nursing and health promotion practice: the creation of victims and winners in a political context.' *Journal of Advanced Nursing*, 19: 465–8.

Caraher, M. (1995) 'Nursing and health education: victim blaming.' *British Journal of Nursing*, 4 (29): 1190–213.

Carey, M.A. (1994) 'The group effect in focus groups: planning, implementing, and interpreting focus group research', in Morse, J. (ed.) *Critical Issues in Qualitative Research Methods*, Thousand Oaks, CA: Sage.

Carey, P. (2000) 'Community health and empowerment', in Kerr, J. (ed.) *Community Health Promotion*, London: Bailliere Tindall.

Carlisle, S. (2000) 'Health promotion, advocacy and health inequalities: a conceptual framework.' *Health Promotion International*, 15 (4): 369–76.

Cartmell, R. and Coles, A. (2000) 'Informed choice in cancer pain: empowering the patient.' *British Journal of Community Nursing*, 5 (11): 560–3.

Casey, D. (2007) 'Using action research to change health-promoting practice.' *Nursing and Health Sciences*, 9: 5–13.

Catford, J. and Nutbeam, D. (1984) 'Towards a definition of health education and health promotion.' *Health Education Journal*, 43 (2 and 3): 38.

Chambers, R., Boath, E. and Chambers, S. (2002) 'Young people's and professionals' views about ways to reduce teenage pregnancy rates: to agree or not agree.' *The Journal of Family Planning and Reproductive Health Care*, 29 (2): 85–90.

Chapman, V. and Slavin, H. (1985) 'The application of models of health education to health visitor training and practice.' First International Conference of Health Education in Nursing, Health Visiting and Midwifery, Harrogate.

Charles, C., Gafni, A. and Whelan, T. (1997) 'Shared decision-making in the medical encounter: what does it mean? (or it takes at least two to tango).' *Social Science & Medicine*, 44 (5): 681–92.

Charles, C.A., Whelan, T., Gafni, A., Willan, A. and Farrell, S. (2003) 'Shared treatment decision-making: what does it mean to physicians?' *Journal of Clinical Oncology*, 21 (5): 932–6.

Chavasse, J.M. (1992) 'Editorial: new dimensions of empowerment in nursing – and challenges.' *Journal of Advanced Nursing*, 17: 1–2.

Cleland, V.S. (1967) 'The use of existing theories.' *Nursing Research*, 16 (2): 118–21.

Cooper, H., Arber, S., Fee, L. and Ginn, J. (1999) *The Influence of Social Support and Social Capital on Health: a review and analysis of British data*, London: Health Education Authority.

Cork, M. (1990) 'Approaches to health promotion.' *Midwife, Health Visitor and Community Nurse*, 26 (5): 169–73.

Cormack, D.F.S. and Reynolds, W. (1992) 'Criteria for evaluating the clinical and practical utility of models used by nurses.' *Journal of Advanced Nursing*, 17: 1472–8.

Coutts, L.C. and Hardy, L.K. (1985) *Teaching for Health: the nurse as health educator*, Edinburgh: Churchill Livingstone.

Crawford, R. (1977) 'You are dangerous to your health: the ideology of victim blaming.' *International Journal of Health Services*, 7 (4): 663–80.

Crawford, R. (1980) 'Healthism and the medicalization of everyday life.' *International Journal of Health Services*, 10 (3): 365–88.

Cribb, A. (1993) 'Health promotion: a human science', in Wilson-Barnett, J. and Macleod Clark, J. (eds) *Research in health promotion and nursing*, Basingstoke: Macmillan, 29–35.

Cribb, A. and Duncan, P. (2001) *Health Promotion and Professional Ethics*, Oxford: Blackwell Science.

Crisp, B.R., Swerissen, H. and Duckett, S.J. (2000) 'Four approaches to capacity building in health: consequences for measurement and accountability.' *Health Promotion International*, 15 (2): 99–107.

Croft, S. and Beresford, P. (1992) 'The politics of participation.' *Critical Social Policy*, 12 (2): 20–44.

Cross, R. (2005) 'Accident and emergency nurses' attitudes towards health promotion.' *Journal of Advanced Nursing*, 51 (5): 474–83.

Crossley, M.L. (2001) 'Rethinking psychological approaches towards health promotion.' *Psychology and Health*, 16: 161–77.

Crotty, M. (1996) *Phenomenology and Nursing Research*, South Melbourne: Churchill Livingstone.

David, J., Zakus, L. and Lysack, C. L. (1998) 'Revisiting community participation.' *Health Policy and Planning*, 13 (1): 1–12.

Davis, S.M. (1995) 'An investigation into nurses' understanding of health education and health promotion within a neuro-rehabilitation setting.' *Journal of Advanced Nursing*, 21: 951–9

Delaney, F.G. (1994) 'Nursing and health promotion: conceptual concerns.' *Journal of Advanced Nursing*, 20: 828–35.

Department of Health (1976) *Prevention and Health: everybody's business*, London: HMSO.

Department of Health (1989) *A Strategy for Nursing*, London: Department of Health Nursing Division.

Department of Health (1992) *The Health of the Nation: a strategy for health in England*, London: HMSO.

Department of Health (1993) *Targeting Practice: the contribution of nurses, midwives and health visitors. The health of the nation*, London: HMSO.

Department of Health (1999a) *Saving Lives: our healthier nation*, London: HMSO.

Department of Health (1999b) *Making a Difference: strengthening the nursing, midwifery and health visiting contribution to health and healthcare*, London: HMSO.

Department of Health (2000) *The NHS Plan: a plan for investment, a plan for reform*, London: HMSO.

Department of Health (2001a) *The Expert Patient: a new approach to chronic disease management for the 21st century*, London: Department of Health.

Department of Health (2001b) *The Health Visitor and School Nurse Development Programme. Health visitor practice development resource pack*, London: Department of Health.

Department of Health (2002a) *Patient Advice and Liaison Service*, London: Department of Health.

Department of Health (2002b) *Tackling Health Inequalities: summary of the cross-cutting review*, London: Department of Health.

Department of Health (2003) *Liberating the Talents: helping Primary Care Trusts and nurses deliver the NHS Plan*, London: HMSO.

Department of Health (2004a) *Choosing Health: making healthy choices easier*, London: Department of Health.

Department of Health (2004b) *Better Information, Better Choices, Better Health: putting information at the centre of health*. www.dh.gov.uk/ (accessed 10 November 2007).

Department of Health (2004c) *Patient and Public Involvement in Health: the evidence of policy implementation*, London: Department of Health.

Department of Health (2005) *Long-term Conditions Information Strategy: supporting the national service framework for long-term conditions*, London: Department of Health.

Department of Health (2006a) *Our Health, Our Care, Our Say: a new direction for community services*, London: Stationery Office.

Department of Health (2006b) *Benchmarks for Promoting Health*, London: Department of Health.

Des Jarlais, D.C. and Friedman, S.R. (1987) 'HIV infection among intravenous drug users: epidemiology and risk reduction.' *AIDS*, 1: 67–76.

Devine, A. (1993) 'Empowering the patient to control post-operative pain.' *British Journal of Theatre Nursing*, 3 (3): 11–12, 29–30.

Dickoff, J. and James, P. (1968) 'A theory of theories: a position paper.' *Nursing Research*, 17 (3): 197–203.

Dickoff, J., James, P. and Wiedenbach, E. (1968) 'Theory in a practice discipline.' *Nursing Research*, 17 (5): 415–35.

DiClemente, C.C. (2005) 'A premature obituary for the transtheoretical model: a response to West.' *Society for the Study of Addiction*, 100: 1046–50.

Dines, A. and Cribb, A. (1993) 'What is health promotion?' in Dines, A. and Cribb, A. (eds) *Health promotion: concepts and practice*, Oxford: Blackwell.

Dinham, A. (2005) 'Empowered or over-powered? The real experience of local participation in the UK's New Deal for Communities.' *Community Development Journal*, 40 (3): 301–12.

Dixon, J. and Sindall, C. (1994) 'Applying logics of change to the evaluation for community development in health promotion.' *Health Promotion International*, 9 (4): 297–309.

Donaldson, S.K. and Crowley, D.M. (1978) 'The discipline of nursing.' *Nursing Outlook*, 26 (2): 113–20.

Donovan, J.L. and Blake, D.R. (1992) 'Patient non-compliance: deviance or reasoned decision-making?' *Social Science and Medicine*, 34 (5): 507–13.

Dooris, M. (2004) 'Joining up settings for health: a valuable investment for strategic partnerships?' *Critical Public Health*, 14 (1): 49–61.

Dooris, M. (2005) 'Healthy settings: challenges to generating evidence of effectiveness.' *Health Promotion International*, 21 (1): 55–65.

Dooris, M. and Hunter, D.J. (2007) 'Organisations and settings for promoting public health', in Lloyd, C.E., Handsley, S., Douglas, J., Earle, S. and Spurr, S. (eds) *Policy and practice in promoting public health*. London: Sage.

Dorn, N. (1981) 'Collaborative work on health education: first working paper on types of health education.' ISDD.

Doty, R.E. (1996) 'Alternative theoretical perspectives: essential knowledge for the advanced practice nurse in the promotion of rural family health.' *Clinical Nurse Specialist*, 10 (5): 217–19.

Douglas, M. (1982) 'Introduction to grid/group analysis', in Douglas, M. (ed.) *Essays in the Sociology of Perception*, London: Routledge & Kegan Paul.

Downie, R.S., Fyfe, C. and Tannahill, A. (1990) *Health Promotion: models and values*, Oxford: Oxford University Press.

Downie, R.S., Tannahill, C. and Tannahill, A. (1996) *Health Promotion: models and values* (2nd edn), Oxford: Oxford University Press.

Draper, P. (1983) 'Tackling the disease of ignorance.' *Self Health*, 1: 23–5.

Draper, P., Griffiths, J., Dennis, J. and Popay, J. (1980) 'Three types of health education.' *British Medical Journal*, 16 August: 493–5.

Earle, S. (2007) 'Promoting public health: exploring the issues', in Earle, S., Lloyd, C.E., Sidell, M. and Spurr, S. (eds) *Theory and Research in Promoting Public Health*, London: Sage: 1–36.

Earp, J.A. and Ennett, S.T. (1991) 'Conceptual models for health education research and practice.' *Health Education Research*, 6 (2): 163–71.

Edgren, L. (1998) 'Co-production: an approach to cardiac rehabilitation from a service management perspective.' *Journal of Nursing Management*, 6: 77–85.

Eggleston, K.S., Coker, A.L., Prabhu Das, I., Cordray, S.T. and Luchok, K.J. (2007) 'Understanding barriers for adherence to follow-up care for abnormal pap tests.' *Journal of Women's Health*, 6 (3): 311–30.

Ellis, R. (1968) 'Characteristics of significant theories.' *Nursing Research*, 17 (5): 217–22.

Elliston, K. and Wilkinson, J. (2004) *Public Health Skills in Nursing Audit Report for Plymouth: building public health through nursing*, Plymouth: Plymouth NHS Teaching Primary Care Trust.

Elrod, C.S. (2007) 'Patient adherence to self-monitoring recommendations taught in extended phase I cardiac rehabilitation.' *Cardiopulmonary Physical Therapy Journal*, 18 (1): 3–14.

Elwyn, G., Edwards, A., Gwyn, R. and Grol, R. (1999) 'Towards a feasible model for shared decision-making: focus group study with general practice registrars.' *BMJ*, 310, 18 September: 753–6.

Elwyn, G., Edwards, A., Kinnnersley, P. and Grol, R. (2000) 'Shared decision-making and the concept of equipoise: the competences of involving patients in healthcare choices.' *British Journal of General Practice*, 50: 892–7.

Epp, J. (1987) 'Achieving health for all: a framework for health promotion.' *Health Promotion*, 1 (4): 419–28.

Ewles, L. and Shipster, P. (1984) *One to One Health Education*, London: South East Thames Regional Health Authority.

Ewles, L. and Simnett, I. (1999) *Promoting Health: a practical guide* (4th edn), Edinburgh: Bailliere Tindall.

Ewles, L. and Simnett, I. (2003) *Promoting Health: a practical guide* (5th edn), Edinburgh: Bailliere Tindall.

Falk-Rafael, A. (1999) 'The politics of health promotion: influences on public health nursing practice in Ontario, Canada from Nightingale to the nineties.' *Advances in Nursing Science*, 22 (1): 23–39.

Falk-Rafael, A.R., Ward-Griffin, C., Laforet-Fliesser, Y. and Beynon, C. (2004) 'Teaching nursing students to promote the health of communities: a partnership approach.' *Nurse Educator*, 29 (2): 63–7.

Fallding, H. (1971) 'Explanatory theory, analytical theory and the ideal type', in Thompson, E. and Tunstall, J. (eds) *Sociological perspectives*, London: Penguin.

Farrant, W. and Russell, J. (1986) *The Politics of Health Information*, Bedford Way Paper No. 2, London: Institute of Education.

Faulkner, M. (2001) 'Empowerment and disempowerment: models of staff/patient interaction.' *NTResearch*, 6 (6): 936–50.

Fawcett, J. (1991) 'Approaches to knowledge development in nursing.' *The Canadian Journal of Nursing Research*, Winter, 23 (4): 23–34.

Fawcett, J. (1995) *Analysis and Evaluation of Conceptual Models of Nursing* (3rd edn), Philadelphia, PA: F.A. Davis Company.

Feyerabend, P. (1975) *Against Method: outline of an anarchistic theory of knowledge*, London: Humanities Press.

Fielding, P. and Woan, M. (1998) 'In sickness and in health.' *Nursing Times*, 94 (7): 36–7.

Fishbein, M. and Ajzen, I. (1985) *Belief, Attitude, Intention and Behaviours: an introduction to theory and research*, Reading, MA: Addison-Wesley.

Fisher, K.F., Howatt, P.A., Binns, C.W. and Liveris, M. (1986) 'Health education and health promotion: an Australian perspective.' *Health Education Journal*, 45 (2): 95–8.

Flanagan, J. (1954) 'The critical incident technique.' *Psychological Bulletin*, 51 (4): 327–58.

Flynn, J.B. and Giffin, P.A. (1984) 'Health promotion in acute settings.' *Nursing Clinics of North America*, 19 (2): 239–250.

Foster, M.C. and Mayall, B. (1990) 'Health visitors as educators.' *Journal of Advanced Nursing*, 15: 286–92.

Frankish C.J. and Green, L.W. (1994) 'Organisational and community change as the social scientific basis for disease prevention and health promotion policy.' *Advances in Medical Sociology*, 4: 209–33.

Franzkowiak, P. and Wenzel, E. (1994) 'AIDS health promotion for youth: conceptual framework and practical implications.' *Health Promotion International*, 9 (2): 119–35.

French, J. (1985) 'To educate or to promote health.' *Health Education Journal*, 44 (3): 115–16.

French, J. (1990) 'Boundaries and horizons: the role of health education within health promotion.' *Health Education Journal*, 49 (1): 7–10.

French, J. and Adams, L. (1986) 'From analysis to synthesis: theories of health education.' *Health Education Journal*, 45 (2): 71–4.

French, J. and Adams, L. (1988) 'Muddled modelling.' *Monitor*, Spring, 76: 14–15.

Freudenberg, N. (1984/5) 'Training health educators for social change.' *International Quarterly of Community Health Education*, 5 (1): 37–52.

Freudenberg, N., Eng, E., Flay, B., Parcal, G., Rogers, T. and Wallerstein, N. (1995) 'Strengthening individual and community capacity to prevent disease and promote health: in search of relevant theories and principles.' *Health in Education Quarterly*, 22 (3): 290–306.

Galvin, K.T. (1992) 'A critical review of the Health Belief Model in relation to cigarette smoking behaviour.' *Journal of Clinical Nursing*, 1: 13–18.

Gastaldo, D. (1997) 'Is health education good for you? Re-thinking health education through the concept of bio-power', in Peterson, A. and Bunton, R. (eds) *Foucault: health and medicine*, London: Routledge.

Gibson, A. (2007) 'Does social capital have a role to play in the health of communities?' in Douglas, J., Earle, S., Handsley, S., Llloyd, C.E. and Spurr, S. (eds) *A Reader in Promoting Public Health*, London: Sage.

Gibson, C.H. (1991) 'A concept analysis of empowerment.' *Journal of Advanced Nursing*, 16: 354–61.

Gilbert, T. (1995) 'Nursing: empowerment and the problem of power.' *Journal of Advanced Nursing*, 21: 865–71.

Gilbert, T. (2001) 'Empowerment: issues, tensions and conflicts', Internal publication, Cambridge: Homerton School of Health Studies.

Gilchrist, A. (2007) 'Community development and networking for health', in Orme, J., Powell, J., Taylor, P. and Grey, M. (eds) *Public Health for the 21st century: new perspectives on policy, participation and practice* (2nd edn), Maidenhead: McGraw-Hill/Open University Press.

Giles, M., Liddell, C. and Bydawell, M. (2005) 'Condom use in African adolescents: the role of individual and group factors.' *AIDS Care*, August, 19 (6): 729–39.

Gomm, R. (1993) 'Issues of power in health and welfare', in Walmsley, J., Reynolds, J., Shakespeare, P. and Woolfe, R. (eds) *Health, Welfare and Practice: reflecting on roles and relationships*, London: Sage.

Gonser, P. and McGuiness, T.M. (2001) 'Theoretical underpinnings of health promotion in acute care.' *Nurse Practitioner Forum*, 12 (3): 147–50.

Goold, P.C., Bustard, S., Ferguson, E., Carlin, E.M., Neal, K. and Bowman, C.A. (2006) 'Pilot study in the development of an Interactive Multimedia Learning Environment for sexual health interventions: a focus group approach.' *Health Education Research*, 21 (1): 15–25.

Gott, M. and O'Brien, M. (1990a) 'Attitudes and beliefs in health promotion.' *Nursing Standard*, 5 (2): 30–2.

Gott, M. and O'Brien, M. (1990b) 'The role of the nurse in health promotion.' *Health Promotion International*, 5 (2): 137–43.

Gottlieb, L. (1992) 'Nurses are not heard in the health promotion movement.' *Canadian Journal of Nursing Research*, 24 (4): 1–2.

Green, L.W. and Raeburn, J.M. (1988) 'Health promotion. What is it? What will it become?' *Health Promotion*, 3 (2): 151–9.

Green, L.W. and Kreuter, M.W. (1990) 'Health promotion as a public health strategy for the 1990s.' *Annual Review of Public Health*, 11: 319–34.

Greenberg, J.S. (1978) 'Health education as freeing.' *Health Education*, March/ April: 20–1.

Greener, J. and Grimshaw, J. (1996) 'Using meta-analysis to summarise evidence within systematic reviews.' *Nurse Researcher*, 4 (1): 27–38.

Griffiths, W. (1972) 'Health education: philosophy, goals, methods, needs and consequences.' *Health Education Monographs*, 31: 7–11.

Groene, O. (2006) *Implementing Health and Promotion in Hospitals: manual and self-assessment forms*, Copenhagen: WHO Europe.

Guba, E.G. and Lincoln, Y.S. (1989) *Fourth Generation Evaluation*, Sage: London.

Hagquist, C. and Starrin, B. (1997) 'Health education in schools: from information to empowerment models.' *Health Promotion International*, 12 (3): 225–32.

Hall, G. (2006) 'Drug concordance and disease control.' *Practice Nurse*, 32 (10): 35–8.

Halpern, D., Bates, C., Beals, G. and Heathfield, A. (2004) *Personal Responsibility and Changing Behaviour: the state of knowledge and its implications for public policy*, London: UK Prime Minister's Strategy Unit, Cabinet Office.

Hamer, L. and Easton, N. (2002) *Community strategies and health improvement: a review of policy and practice*, London: Health Development Agency.

Hancock, T. (1999) 'Creating health and health promoting hospitals: a worthy challenge for the twenty-first century.' *International Journal of Health Care Quality Assurance, incorporating Leadership in Health Services*, 12 (2): viii–xix.

Handsley, S. (2007a) 'The potential for promoting health at a local level: community strategies and health improvement', in Lloyd, C.E., Handsley, S., Douglas, J., Earle, S. and Spurr, S. (eds) *Policy and Practice in Promoting Public Health*, London: Sage.

Handsley, S. (2007b) 'Part V. Promoting health at a local level. Introduction', in Douglas, J., Earle, S., Handsley, S., Lloyd, C.E. and Spurr, S. (eds) *A Reader in Promoting Public Health*, London: Sage.

Handsley, S. (2007c) 'Community involvement and civic engagement in multi-disciplinary public health', in Lloyd, C.E., Handsley, S., Douglas, J., Earle, S. and Spurr, S. (eds) *Policy and Practice in Promoting Public Health*. London: Sage.

Hart, N. (1985) *The Sociology of Health and Medicine*, Ormskirk: Causeway Books.

Hashagen, S. and Paxton, S. (2007) 'Frameworks for evaluation of community health and well-being work', in Orme, J., Powell, J., Taylor, P. and Grey, M. (eds) *Public Health for the 21st century: new perspectives on policy, participation and practice* (2nd edn), Maidenhead: McGraw-Hill/Open University Press.

Hawe, P., King, L., Noort, M., Gifford, S.M. and Lloyd, B. (1998) 'Working invisibly: health workers talk about capacity-building in health promotion.' *Health Promotion International*, 13 (4): 285–95.

Health Development Agency (2003) *The Working Partnership. Book 1: introduction*, London: Health Development Agency.

Health Education Authority (1993) *Health Promoting Hospitals: principles and practice*, London: Health Education Authority.

Health Education Journal (1990) 49 (1).

Henderson, V. (1970) 'The concept of nursing.' *Journal of Advanced Nursing*, 3: 113–30.

Henwood, F., Wyatt, S., Hart, A. and Smith, J. (2003) '"Ignorance is bliss sometimes": constraints on the emergence of the "informed patient" in the changing landscapes of health information.' *Sociology of Health & Illness*, 25 (6): 589–607.

Hewitt-Taylor, J. (2004) 'Challenging the balance of power: patient empowerment.' *Nursing Standard*, 18 (22): 33–7.

Hills, M. (1998) 'Student experiences of nursing health promotion practice in hospital settings.' *Nursing Inquiry*, 5: 164–73.

Hills, P. (1979) *Teaching and Learning as a Communication Process*, Croom Helm: London.

Hobden, A. (2006a) 'Concordance: a widely used term, but what does it mean?' *British Journal of Community Nursing*, 11 (6): 257–60.

Hobden, A. (2006b) 'Strategies to promote concordance within consultations.' *British Journal of Community Nursing*, 11 (7): 286–9.

Hogg, C. (1999) *Patients, Power and Politics. From patients to citizens*, London: Sage Publications.

Holloway, I. and Wheeler, S. (1996) *Qualitative Research for Nurses*, Oxford: Blackwell.

Holt, M. and Warne, T. (2007) 'The educational and practice tensions in preparing pre-registration nurses to become future health promoters: a small scale explorative study.' *Nurse Education Today*, 7: 373–80.

Hopson, B. and Scally, M. (1981) *Lifeskills Teaching*, London: McGraw-Hill.

Horner, J.S. (1980) 'Health education and public policy in the United Kingdom.' *Community Medicine*, 2: 229–35.

Hornsey, E. (1982) 'Health education in pre-retirement education: a question of relevance.' *Health Education Journal*, 41 (4): 107–13.

Hsiao, Y., Chen, M., Gau, Y., Hung, L., Chang, S. and Tsai, H. (2005) 'Short-term effects of a health promotion course for Taiwanese nursing students.' *Public Health Nursing*, 22 (1): 74–81.

Humphries, B. (1996) 'Contradictions in the culture of empowerment', in Humphries, B. (ed.) *Critical perspectives on empowerment*. Birmingham: Venture Press.

Hycner, R.H. (1985) 'Some guidelines for phenemenological analysis of interview data.' *Human Studies*, 8: 279–303.

International Council of Nurses (2004) *Position Statement: scope of nursing practice*. Geneva: International Council of Nurses.

Irvine, F. (2005) 'Exploring district nursing competencies in health promotion: the use of the Delphi technique.' *Journal of Clinical Nursing*, 14: 965–75.

Jack, R. (1995a) 'Empowerment in community care', in Jack, R. (ed.) *Empowerment in community care*, London: Chapman & Hall.

Jack, R. (1995b) 'Introduction', in Jack, R. (ed.) *Empowerment in community care*, London: Chapman & Hall.

Jacob, F. (1996) 'Empowerment: a critique.' *British Journal of Community Health Nursing*, 1: 449–553.

Jary, D. and Jary, J. (1991) *Collins Dictionary of Sociology*, Glasgow: Harper Collins.

Johnson, A. and Baum, F. (2001) 'Health promoting hospitals: a typology of different organisational approaches to health promotion.' *Health Promotion International*, 16 (3): 281–7.

Johnson, D.E. (1968) 'Theory in nursing: borrowed and unique.' *Nursing Research*, 17 (3): 206–9.

Johnson, D.E. (1974) 'Development of theory: a requisite for nursing as a primary health profession.' *Nursing Research*, 23 (5): 372–7.

Johnson, J.L. (2000) 'The health care institution as a setting for health promotion', in Poland, B.D., Green, L.W. and Rootman, I. (eds) *Settings for Health Promotion: linking theory and practice*. London: Sage.

Jones, K. (1993) 'Opportunities for health education: an analysis of nurse–client interactions in acute areas', in Wilson-Barnett, J. and Macleod Clark, J. (eds) *Research in Health Promotion and Nursing*, Basingstoke: Macmillan.

Jones, L. (1997) 'Health promotion and public policy', in Jones, L. and Sidell, M. (eds) *The Challenge of Promoting Health: exploration and action*. Hampshire: Macmillan/Open University: 91–111.

Jones, L. and Naidoo, J. (2000) 'Theories and models in health promotion', in Katz, J., Peberdy, A. and Douglas, J. (eds) *Promoting health: knowledge and practice* (2nd edn), Hampshire: Open University/Palgrave.

Jones, L. and Douglas, J. (2000) 'The rise of health promotion', in Katz, J., Peberdy, A. and Douglas, J. (eds) *Promoting Health: knowledge and practice* (2nd edn), Hampshire: Open University/Palgrave.

Jones, L.D. (1990) 'Working with drug users to prevent the spread of HIV: the application of an analytical framework to a range of programmes.' *Health Education research*, 5 (1): 5–16.

Jones, L.J. (1994) *The Social Context of Health and Health Work*, Hampshire: Macmillan.

Jowett, S. (1992) 'A health model for community nursing.' *Nursing Standard*, 6 (25): 33–5.

Judd, C.M., Smith, E.R. and Kidder, L.M. (1991) *Research Methods in Social Relations* (6th edn), Fort Worth: Holt, Rhinehart & Winston.

Kasl, S. and Cobb, S. (1966) 'Health behaviour, illness behaviour.' *Archives of Environmental Health*, 12: 246–66.

Kawachi, I., Kennedy, B.P., Lochner, K., Prothrow-Smith, S.M. and Prothrow-Smith, D. (1997) 'Social capital, income inequality and mortality.' *American Journal of Public Health*, 87 (9): 1491–8.

Keeley-Robinson, Y. (1984) 'Adult education issues for health education: a review and annotated bibliography', Occasional Paper No. 1. Institute for Health Studies, Hull University.

Kelly, K. and Abraham, C. (2007) 'Health promotion for people aged over 65 years in hospitals: nurses' perceptions about their role.' *Journal of Clinical Nursing*, 16: 569–79.

Kemm, J. and Close, A. (1995) *Health Promotion: theory and practice*, Basingstoke: Macmillan.

Kemshall, H. and Littlechild, R. (2000) *User Involvement and Participation in Social Care: research informing practice*, London: Jessica Kingsley.

221

Kendall, S. (1998) 'Introduction', in Kendall, S. (ed.) *Health and Empowerment: research and practice*. London: Arnold.

Kerlinger, F.N. (1964) *Foundations of Behavioural Research*, New York: Holt, Rhinehart & Winston.

Kettunen, T., Poskiparta, M. and Liimutainen, L. (2001) 'Empowering counselling – a case study: nurse–patient encounter in a hospital.' *Health Education Research*, 16 (2): 227–38.

Keyes, L. (1972) 'Health education in perspective: an overview.' *Health Education Monographs*, 31: 13–17.

Kickham, N. and Rushmere, A. (1998) 'Alliance in secondary care: health promoting hospitals', in Scriven, A. (ed.) *Alliances in Health Promotion: theory and practice*, Basingstoke: Macmillan.

Kieffer, C.H. (1984) 'Citizen empowerment: a developmental perspective.' *Prevention in human services*, 3: 9–36.

Kiger, A.M. (2004) *Teaching for Health* (3rd edn), Edinburgh: Churchill Livingstone.

King, P.M. (1994) 'Health promotion: the emerging frontier in nursing.' *Journal of Advanced Nursing*, 20: 209– 18.

Kitzinger, J. (1995) 'Introducing focus groups.' *British Medical Journal*, 311: 299–302.

Kuokkanen, L. and Leino-Kilpi, H. (2000) 'Power and empowerment in nursing: three theoretical approaches.' *Journal of Advanced Nursing*, 31 (1): 235–41.

Kuss, T., Proulx-Giroud, L., Lovitt, S., Katz, C.B. and Kennelly, P. (1997) 'A public health nursing model.' *Public Health Nursing*, 14 (2): 81–91.

Labonte, R. (1989) 'Community and professional empowerment.' *The Canadian Nurse*, 85 (3): 23–8.

Labonte, R. (1993) 'Community development and partnerships.' *Canadian Journal of Public Health*, 84 (4): 237–40.

Lalonde, M. (1974) 'A new perspective on the health of Canadians: a working document.' Government of Canada.

Lask, S. (1987) 'Beliefs and behaviour in health education.' *Nursing*, 18: 681–3.

Latter, S. (1993) 'Health education and health promotion in acute ward settings: nurses' perceptions and practice', in Wilson-Barnett, J. and Macleod Clark, J. (eds) *Research in health promotion and nursing*, Basingstoke: Macmillan.

Latter, S. (1998) 'Health promotion in the acute setting: the case for empowering nurses', in Kendall, S. (ed.) *Health and Empowerment: research and practice*. London: Arnold.

Latter, S. (2001) 'The potential for health promotion in hospital nursing practice', in Scriven, A. and Orme, J. (eds) *Health Promotion: professional perspectives* (2nd edn). Basingstoke: Palgrave.

Latter, S., Macleod Clark, J., Wilson-Barnett, J. and Maben, J. (1992) 'Health education in nursing: perceptions of practice in acute settings.' *Journal of Advanced Nursing*, 17: 164–72.

Laudan, L. (1981) 'A problem solving approach to scientific progress', in Hacking, I. (ed.) *Scientific Revolutions*, Oxford: Oxford University Press.

Laverack, G. (2005) *Public Health: power, empowerment and professional practice*, Basingstoke: Palgrave Macmillan.

Laverack, G. and Wallerstein, N. (2001) 'Measuring community empowerment: a fresh look at organizational domains.' *Health Promotion International*, 16 (2): 179–85.

Lewin, D. and Piper, S.M. (2007) 'Patient empowerment within a coronary care unit.' *Intensive and Critical Care Nursing*, 23: 81–90.

Lincoln, Y.S. and Guba, E.G. (1985) *Naturalistic Inquiry*, London: Sage.

Liverpool Declaration on the Right to Health (1988) World Health Organization Healthy Cities Project, Liverpool: Healthy Cities Inter-Sectoral Committee.

Loft, M., McWilliam, C. and Ward-Griffin, C. (2003) 'Patient empowerment after total hip and knee replacement.' *Orthopaedic Nursing*, 22 (1): 42–7.

Lovemore, L. and Dann, K.L. (2002) 'Empowerment in nursing: the role of philosophical and psychological factors.' *Nursing Philosophy*, 3: 234–9.

Lowenberg, J.S. (1995) 'Health promotion and the ideology of choice.' *Public Health Nursing*, 12 (5): 319–23.

Lupton, L. (1997) 'Foucault and the medicalisation critique', in Peterson, A. and Bunton, R. (eds) *Foucault: health and medicine*, London: Routledge.

Maben, J.M. and Macleod Clark, J. (1995) 'Health promotion: a concept analysis.' *Journal of Advanced Nursing*, 22: 1158–65.

Maben, J., Latter, S., Macleod Clark, J. and Wilson-Barnett, J. (1993) 'The organization of care: its influence on health education practice on acute wards.' *Journal of Clinical Nursing*, 2: 355–62.

McBean, S. (1992) 'Promoting positive health.' *Primary Health Care*, 2 (4): 10–13.

McBride, A. (1994) 'Health promotion in hospitals: the attitudes, beliefs and practices of hospital nurses.' *Journal of Advanced Nursing*, 20: 92–100.

McBride, A. (1995) *Health Promotion in Hospital: a practical handbook for nurses*, London: Scutari.

McDonald, E. (1998) 'The role of Project 2000 educated nurses in health promotion within the hospital setting.' *Nurse Education Today*, 18: 213–20.

McEwan, R. and Bhopal, R. (1991) 'HIV/AIDS health promotion for young people: a review of theory, principles and practice.' HIV/AIDS and Sexual Health Programme Paper 12. London: HEA.

Macleod Clark, J. and Webb, P. (1985) 'Health education: a basis for professional practice.' *Nurse Education Today*, 5: 210–14.

Macleod Clark, J. and Maben, J. (1998) 'Health promotion: perceptions of Project 2000 educated nurses.' *Health Education Research*, 13 (2): 185–96.

Macleod Clark, J., Wilson-Barnet, T.J. and Latter, S. (1991) *Health Education in Nursing Project: results of a national survey on service nurse perceptions of health education practice in acute ward settings*, London: King's College.

Macleod Clark, J., Maben, J. and Jones, K. (1996) *Project 2000: perceptions of the philosophy and practice of nursing*. www.enb.org.uk/rh17.htm (accessed 2007).

McLeroy, K.R., Bibeau, D., Steckler, A. and Glanz, K. (1988) 'An ecological perspective on health promotion programmes.' *Health Education Quarterly*, 15 (4): 351–77.

McLeroy, K.R., Steckler, A.B., Goodman, R.M. and Burdine, J.N. (1992) 'Health education research: theory and practice – future directions.' *Health Education Research*, 7: 1–8.

McQueen, D., White, P.D., Fuller, R. and Sharpe, M.C. (2002) 'Discomfort of patient power.' *British Medical Journal*, May 18, 324: 1214.

Maidwell, A. (1996) 'The role of the surgical nurse as a health promoter.' *British Journal of Nursing*, 5 (15): 898–904.

Malin, N. and Teasdale, K. (1991) 'Caring versus empowerment; considerations for nursing practice.' *Journal of Advanced Nursing*, 16: 657–62.

Marriner-Tomey, A. (1989) *Nursing Theorists and their Work* (2nd edn), St Louis, MO: Mosby.

Massey, D.E. and Carnell, E.B. (1987) 'Health education in school: negotiation or prescription?' *Monitor*, Summer, 74: 10–12.

May, C. (1992) 'Nursing work, nurses' knowledge, and the subjectification of the patient.' *Sociology of Health and Illness*, 14 (4): 472–87.

May, K.A. (1991) 'Interview techniques in qualitative research: concerns and challenges', in Morse, J.M. (ed.) *Qualitative Nursing Research: a contemporary dialogue*, London: Sage.

Mayer, J.P., Soweid, R., Dabney, S., Brownson, C., Goodman, R.M. and Brownson, R.C. (1998) 'Practices of successful community coalitions: a multiple case study.' *American Journal of Health Behavior*, 22 (5): 368–77.

Meleis, A.I. (1985) *Theoretical Nursing: development and progress*, Philadelphia, PA: Lippincott.

Meleis, A.I. (2007) *Theoretical Nursing: development and progress* (4th edn), Philadelphia, PA: Lippincott.

Miles, M.B. and Huberman, A.M. (1994) *Qualitative Data Analysis: an expanded sourcebook*, London: Sage.

Miller, S. (1997) 'Multiple paradigms for nursing: post modern feminism', in Thorne, S.E. and Hayes, V.E. (eds) *Nursing Praxis: knowledge and action*. Thousand Oaks, CA: Sage.

Mills, C.W. (1943) 'The professional ideology of social pathologists.' *American Journal of Sociology*, 49 (2): 165–80.

Mills, C.W. (1959) *The Sociological Imagination*, London: Oxford University Press.

Ministry of Health (1964) *Health Education. Report of a joint committee of the Central and Scottish Health Services Councils*, London: HMSO.

Ministry of Health (2001) *The Primary Health Care Strategy*, Ministry of Health. Wellington: New Zealand.

Minkler, M. (1989) 'Health education, health promotion and the open society: an historical perspective.' *Health Education Quarterly*, 16 (1): 17–30.

Mitchell, G.J. (1992) 'Specifying the knowledge of theory in practice.' *Nursing Science Quarterly*, 5 (1): 6–7.

Mitchell, J. (1982) 'Looking after ourselves: an individual responsibility.' *Royal Society of Health Journal*, (4): 169–73.

Mitchenson, S. (1995) 'A review of health promotion and health beliefs of traditional and Project 2000 student nurses.' *Journal of Advanced Nursing*, 21: 356–63.

Mitre, J.C., Alexander, J.E. and Keller, S.L. (1998) 'Patricia Benner: from novice to expert: excellence and power in clinical nursing practice', in Marriner Tomey, A. and Alligood, M.R. (eds) *Nursing Theorists and Their Work* (4th edn), St Louis, MO: Mosby.

Mittelmark, M.B. (2007) 'Promoting social responsibility for health: health impact assessment and healthy public policy at the community level', in Douglas, J., Earle, S., Handsley, S., Lloyd, C.E. and Spurr, S. (eds) *A Reader in Promoting Public Health*, London: Sage.

Morgan, I.S. and Marsh, G.W. (1998) 'Historic and future health promotion contexts for nursing.' *Journal of Nursing Scholarship*, 30 (4): 379–83.

Morrow, V. (1999) 'Conceptualising social capital in relation to the well-being of children and young people: a critical review.' *The Sociological Review*, 47 (4): 744–65.

Morse, J.M. and Field, P.A. (1985) *Nursing Research: the application of qualitative approaches*, London: Croom Helm.

Mosby's Medical, Nursing, & Allied Health Dictionary (2002) (6th edn), Mosby.

Muntainer, C., Lynch, J. and Smith, G.D. (2000) 'Social capital and the third way in public health.' *Critical Public Health*, 10 (2): 107–23.

Naidoo, J. and Wills, J. (2000) *Health Promotion: foundations for practice* (2nd edn), London: Bailliére Tindall.

Naidoo, J. and Wills, J. (2005) *Public Health and Health Promotion: developing practice*, London: Bailliére Tindall.

NAM Publications (1999) 'Factsheet 36: Adherence tips', London: National Aids Manual.

National Academy of Sciences (2002) *The Future of the Public's Health in the 21st Century. Committee on Assuring the Health of the Public in the 21st Century*, National Academy of Sciences.

Nelson, D. and Ruth, A. (1998) 'Raising accident awareness in children.' *Managing Clinical Nursing*, 2: 2–4.

NHS Management Executive (1993) *Patient Empowerment*, London: NHS Management Executive.

NHS Management Executive (1994) *Health Promoting Hospitals*, London: NHS Management Executive.

NHSE (1997) *Health Research: what's in it for consumers? First Report of the Standing Advisory Group on Consumer Involvement in the NHS Research and Development Programme*, London: NHSE.

Nightingale, F. (1860) *Notes on Nursing: what it is, and what it is not* (1st American edn), New York: D. Appleton & Company. www.digital.library.upenn.edu/women/nightingale/nursing/html (accessed 27 September 2007).

Noak, H. (1987) 'Concepts of health and health promotion', in Abelin, T., Brzezinski, Z.J. and Carstairs, B.D.L. (eds) *Measurement in Health Promotion and Health Protection*. WHO Regional Publications, European Series No. 22: 5–8.

Norman, I.J., Redfern, S.J., Tomalin, D.A. and Oliver, S. (1992) 'Developing Flanagan's critical incident technique to elicit indicators of high quality and low quality nursing care from patients and nurses.' *Journal of Advanced Nursing*, 17: 590–600.

Northrup, D.T. and Purkis, M.E. (2001) 'Building the science of health promotion practice from a human science perspective.' *Nursing Philosophy*, 2: 62–71.

Norton, L. (1998) 'Health promotion and health education: what role should the nurse adopt in practice?' *Journal of Advanced Nursing*, 28 (6): 1269–75.

Nursing and Midwifery Council (2004a) *Standards of Proficiency for Pre-registration Nursing Education*, London: Nursing and Midwifery Council.

Nursing and Midwifery Council (2004b) *Standards of Proficiency for Specialist Community Public Health Nurses*, London: Nursing and Midwifery Council.

Nursing and Midwifery Council (2004c) *The NMC Code of Professional Conduct: standards for conduct, performance and ethics*, London: Nursing and Midwifery Council.

Nursing Council of New Zealand (2005) *Education Programme Standards for the Registered Nurse Scope of Practice*, Wellington: Nursing Council of New Zealand.

Nutbeam, D. (1984) 'Health education in the National Health Service: the differing perceptions of community physicians and health education officers.' *Health Education Journal*, 43 (4): 115–19.

225

Nutbeam, D. (1986) 'Health promotion glossary.' *Health Promotion*, 1 (1): 113–26.

Nutbeam, D. and Blakey, V. (1990) 'The concept of health promotion and AIDS prevention. A comprehensive and integrated basis for action in the 1990s.' *Health Promotion International*, 5 (3): 233–42.

Nyamwaya, D. (1997) 'Health promotion practice: the need for an integrated and processual approach.' *Health Promotion International*, 12 (3): 179–81.

O'Donnell, M. (1989) 'Definition of health promotion: Part III: expanding the definition.' *American Journal of Health Promotion*, 3 (3): 5.

Orme, J., Powell, J., Taylor, P. and Grey, M. (2007) *Public Health for the 21st Century: new perspectives on policy, participation and practice* (2nd edn), Maidenhead: McGraw-Hill/Open University Press.

Parish, R. (1995) 'Health promotion: rhetoric and reality', in Bunton, R. and Macdonald, G. (eds) *Health Promotion: disciplines and diversity*, London: Routledge.

Parse, R. (1990) 'Editorial. Promotion and prevention: two distinct cosmologies.' *Nursing Science Quarterly*, 3 (3): 101.

Parse, R.R. (1999) 'Nursing science: the transformation of practice.' *Journal of Advanced Nursing*, 30 (6): 1383–7.

Parsloe, P. (1997) 'Everyday choices may be as important as the grand notion.' *Care Plan*, March: 9–12.

Patton, M.L. (1990) *Qualitative Evaluation and Research Methods*, London: Sage.

Pederson, L.L., Wanklin, J.M., Bull, S.B. and Ashley, M.J. (1991) 'A conceptual framework for the roles of legislation and education in reducing exposure to environmental tobacco smoke.' *American Journal of Health Promotion*, 6 (2): 105–11.

Pender, N.J. (1996) *Health Promotion in Nursing Practice* (3rd edn), Stamford, CT: Appleton and Lange.

Peterson, A. (1997) 'Risk, governance and the new public health', in Peterson, A. and Bunton, R. (eds) *Foucault: health and medicine*. London: Routledge.

Philips, J.R. (1977) 'Nursing systems and nursing models.' *Image*, 9 (1): 4–7.

Piper, S.M. (2000) 'Promoting health.' *Nursing Management*, 7 (4): 8–11.

Piper, S.M. (2004) 'An interpretive inquiry testing the relationship between health promotion theory and nursing practice.' Unpublished PhD thesis, Cambridge: Anglia Ruskin University.

Piper, S.M. (2005) 'Health promotion: a practice framework for midwives.' *British Journal of Midwifery*, 13 (5): 284–8.

Piper, S.M. (2007a) 'A qualitative study testing the relationship between health promotion theory and nursing practice.' *Nursing Times*, 103 (6): 34–5.

Piper, S.M. (2007b) 'Health promotion and accident and emergency nursing: theory and practice', in Dolan, B. and Holt, L. (eds) *Accident and Emergency Care* (2nd edn). London: Bailliére Tindall.

Piper, S.M. (2008) 'A qualitative study exploring the relationship between nursing and health promotion language, theory and practice.' *Nurse Education Today*, 28: 186–93.

Piper, S.M. and Brown, P.A. (1998a) 'The theory and practice of health education applied to nursing: a bi-polar approach.' *Journal of Advanced Nursing*, 27: 383–9.

Piper, S.M. and Brown, P.A. (1998b) 'Psychology as a theoretical foundation for health education in nursing: empowerment or social control?' *Nurse Education Today*, 18: 637–41.

Polit, D.F. and Beck C.T. (2006) *Essentials of Nursing Research: methods, appraisal and ulilization* (6th edn), Philadelphia, PA: Lippincott, Williams and Wilkins.

Polit, D.F. and Hungler B.P. (1993) *Essentials of Nursing Research: methods, appraisal and utilization*, Philadelphia, PA: Lippincott.

Pratt, R.J., Robinson, N., Loveday, H.P., Pellowe, C.M., Franks, P.J., Hankins, M. and Loveday, C. (2001) 'Adherence to antiretroviral therapy: appropriate use of self-report in clinical practice.' *HIV Clinical Trials*, 2 (2): 146–59.

Primary Health Care Nursing Innovation Evaluation Team (2007) *The Evaluation of the Eleven Primary Health Care Nursing Innovation Projects: a report to the Ministry of Health by the Primary Health Care Nursing Innovation Evaluation Team.* Wellington: New Zealand.

Prochaska, J.O. and DiClemente, C.C. (1982) 'Transtheoretical therapy: towards a more integrative model of change.' *Psychotherapy, Theory, Research and Practice* 19 (3): 276–88.

Prochaska, J.O., DiClemente, C.C. and Norcross, J.C. (1992) 'In search of how people change: applications to addictive behaviours.' *American Psychologist*, 47 (9): 1102–14.

Putnam, R.D. (2000) *Bowling Alone: the collapse and revival of American community*, London: Simon & Schuster.

Quinn, F. (1995) *The Principles and Practice of Nurse Education* (3rd edn), London: Chapman Hall.

Raphael, D., Steinmetz, B., Renwick, R., Rootman, I., Brown, I., Sehdev, H., Phillips, S. and Smith, T. (1999) 'The community quality of life project: a health promotion approach to understanding communities.' *Health Promotion International*, 14 (3): 197–209.

Rappaport, J. (1984) 'Studies in empowerment: introduction to the issue.' *Prevention in Human Services*, 3: 1–7.

Rawson, D. (1990) *The Language of Theoretical Debate: a brief guide to some of the major terms*, London: South Bank Polytechnic.

Rawson, D. (2002) 'The growth of health promotion theory and its rational reconstruction: lessons from the philosophy of science', in Bunton, R. and Macdonald, G. (eds) *Health Promotion: disciplines and diversity* (2nd edn), London: Routledge.

Rawson, D. and Grigg, C. (1988) 'Purpose and practice in health education. The training and development needs of Health Education Officers.' The summary report of the SHER Project, London: South Bank Polytechnic/Health Education Authority.

Rissel, C. (1994) 'Empowerment: the holy grail of health promotion?' *Health Promotion International*, 9 (1): 39–47.

Robertson, R. (1974) 'Toward the identification of the major axes of sociological analysis', in Rex, J. (ed.) *Approaches to Sociology*, London: Routledge.

Robinson, A. and Miller, M. (1996) 'Making information accessible: developing plain English discharge instructions.' *Journal of Advanced Nursing*, 24: 528–35.

Robinson, S. and Hill, Y. (1998) 'The health promoting nurse.' *Journal of Clinical Nursing*, 7: 232–8.

Robinson, S.E. and Hill, Y. (1999) 'Our healthier hospital? The challenge for nursing.' *Journal of Nursing Management*, 7: 13–17.

Roden, J. (2004) 'Validating the revised health belief model for young families: implications for nurses' health promotion practice.' *Nursing and Health Sciences*, 6: 247–59.

Rodmell, S. and Watt, A. (1986) *The Politics of Health Education*, London: Routledge.

Rodwell, C.M. (1996) 'An analysis of the concept of empowerment.' *Journal of Advanced Nursing*, 23: 305–13.

Rose, N. (1996) 'The death of the social? Re-figuring the territory of government.' *Economy and Society*, 25 (3): 327–56.

Rosen, M.I., Dieckhaus, K., McMahon, T.J., Valdes, B., Petry, N.M., Cramer, J. and Rounsaville, B. (2007) 'Improved adherence with contingency management.' *Aids, Patient Care and STDs*, 21 (1): 30–40.

Rosenstock, I.M., Strecher, V.J. and Becker, M.H. (1988) 'Social learning theory and the health belief model.' *Health Education Quarterly*, 15 (2): 172–83.

Royal College of Nursing (2002) *The Community Approach to Improving Public Health: community nurses and community development*, London: Royal College of Nursing.

Royal College of Nursing (2003) *Defining Nursing*, London: Royal College of Nursing.

Royal College of Nursing (2007) *Nurses as Partners in Delivering Public Health: a paper to support the nursing contribution to public health, developed by an alliance of organisations*, London: Royal College of Nursing.

Rush, K.L. (1997) 'Health promotion ideology and nursing education.' *Journal of Advanced Nursing*, 25: 1292–8.

Rushmere, A. (2000) *Health Promoting Hospitals and Trusts: self assessment and peer review toolkit*. The Wessex Institute for Health Research and Development.

Rutten, A. (1995) 'The implementation of health promotion: a new structural perspective.' *Social Science and Medicine*, 41 (12): 1627–37.

Salmon, P. and Hall, G.M. (2004) 'Patient empowerment or the emperor's new clothes?' *Journal of the Royal Society of Medicine*, 97 (2): 53–6.

Salvage, J. (1990) 'The theory and practice of the "new nursing".' *Nursing Times*, 86 (4): 42–5.

Sapsford, R. and Abbott, P. (1992) *Research Methods for Nurses and the Caring Professions*, Buckingham: Open University Press.

Sawka, C.A., Goel, V., Mahut, C.A., Taylor, G.A. Thiel, E.C., O'Connor, A.M., Ackerman, I., Burt, J.H. and Gort, E.H. (1998) 'Development of a patient decision aid for choice of surgical treatment for breast cancer.' *Health Expectations*, 1: 23–36.

Schutz, A. (1971) 'Concept and theory formation in the social sciences', in Thompson, K. and Tunstall, J. (eds) *Sociological Perspectives*. London: Penguin.

Scriven, A. (2005) 'Promotion health: perspectives, principles, practice', in Scriven, A. (ed.) *Health Promoting Practice: the contribution of nurses and allied health professionals*, Basingstoke: Palgrave Macmillan.

The Secretariat for the Intersectoral Healthy Living network in partnership with the F/P/T Healthy Living Task Group and the F/P/T Advisory Committee on Population Health and Health Security (ACPHHS) (2005) *The Integrated Pan-Canadian Healthy Living Strategy*.

Seedhouse, D. (1986) *Health: the foundations for achievement*, Chichester: John Wiley & Sons.

Seedhouse, D. (1997) *Health Promotion: philosophy, prejudice and practice*, Chichester: Wiley.

Segan, C.J., Borland, R., Greenwood, K.M. (2004) 'What is the right thing at the right time? Interactions between stages and processes of change among smokers who make a quit attempt.' *Health Psychology*, 23 (1): 86–93.

Seymour, M. (1984) 'Health education versus health promotion: a practitioner's view.' *Health Educational Journal*, 43 (2 and 3): 37–8.

Shediac-Rizkallah, M.C. and Bone, L.R. (1998) 'Planning for the sustainability of community-based health programs: conceptual frameworks and future direction for research, practice and policy.' *Health Education Research: Theory and Practice*, 13 (1): 87–108.

Sherman, F.T. (2007) 'Medication nonadherence: a national epidemic among America's seniors.' *Geriatrics*, April, 62 (4): 5–6.

Silva, M.C. (1986) 'Research testing nursing theory: state of the art.' *Advances in Nursing Science*, 9 (1): 1–11.

Silva, M.C. and Rothbart, D. (1984) 'An analysis of changing trends in philosophies of science on nursing theory development and testing.' *Advances in Nursing Science*, January: 1–13.

Skelton, R. (1994) 'Nursing and empowerment: concepts and strategies.' *Journal of Advanced Nursing*, 19: 415–23.

Skybo, T. and Polivka, B. (2006) 'Health promotion model for childhood violence prevention and exposure.' *Journal of Clinical Nursing*, 16: 38–45.

Smith, M. and Cusack, L. (2000) 'The Ottawa Charter – from nursing theory to practice: insights from the area of alcohol and other drugs.' *International Journal of Nursing Practice*, 6: 168–73.

Smith, P., Masterson, A. and Lask, S. (1995a) 'Health and the curriculum: an illuminative evaluation. Part 1: Methodology. *Nurse Education Today*, 15: 245–9.

Smith, P., Masterson, A. and Lask, S. (1995b) 'Health and the curriculum: an illuminative evaluation. Part 2: Methodology. *Nurse Education Today*, 15: 317–22.

Smithies, J. and Webster, G. (undated) 'Community participation.' A paper for the UK healthy cities community participation group.

Snape, D. (2000) 'Concepts of health and the health promoting role of the perioperative nurse.' *British Journal of Perioperative Nursing*. 10 (7): 43–9.

Snee, K. (1991) 'Neighbourhood needs.' *Community Outlook*, February: 38–9.

Sriven, A. (2005) 'Promoting health: perspectives, principles, practice', in Sriven, A. (ed.) *Health Promoting Practice: the contribution of nurses and allied health professionals*, Basingstoke: Palgrave Macmillan.

St Leger, L. (1999) 'Health promotion indicators. Coming out of the maze with a purpose.' *Health Promotion International*, 14 (3): 193–5.

Statutory Instruments (1983) No. 873. *The Nurses, Midwives and Health Visitors Rules Approvals Order 1983*, London: HMSO.

Stewart, D.W. and Shamdasani, P.N. (1990) *Focus Groups: theory and practice*, Newbury Park: Sage.

Stewart, M.J. (1989) 'Nurses' preparedness for health promotion through linkage with mutual-aid self help groups.' *Canadian Journal of Public Health*, March/April, 80: 110–14.

Stokols, D. (1996) 'Translating social ecological theory into guidelines for community health promotion.' *American Journal of Health Promotion*, 10 (4): 282–98.

Streubert, H.J. and Carpenter, D.R. (1999) *Qualitative Research in Nursing: advancing the humanistic imperative*, Philadelphia, PA: Lippincott.

Suppe, F. and Jacox, A.K. (1985) 'The philosophy of science and the development of nursing theory.' *Annual Review of Nursing Research*, 3: 241–67.

Syred, M.E.J. (1981) 'The abdication of the role of health education by hospital nurses.' *Journal of Advanced Nursing*, 6: 27–33.

Tabi, M.M. (2002) 'Community perspective on a model to reduce teenage pregnancy.' *Journal of Advanced Nursing*, 40 (3): 275–84.

Tannahill, A. (1985) 'What is health promotion?' *Health Education Journal*, 44 (4): 167–8.

Tannahill, A. (1990) 'Health education and health promotion: planning for the 1990s.' *Health Education Journal*, 49 (4): 194–8.

Taylor, V. (1990) 'Health education: a theoretical mapping.' *Health Education Journal*, 49 (1): 13–14.

Thomson, P. (1998) 'Application of the planning compass to the nursing curriculum: a tool for health promotion practice.' *Nurse Education Today*, 18: 406–12.

Tomalin, C. (1981) 'On the front line.' *Nursing Mirror*, 11 November: 34–5.

Tones, B.K. (1981) 'Health education: prevention or subversion?' *Royal Society of Health Journal*, 3: 114–17.

Tones, B.K. (1986) 'Health education and the ideology of health promotion: a review of alternative approaches.' *Health Education Research*, 1 (1): 3–12.

Tones, K. (1985) 'Health promotion: a new panacea?' *Journal of the Institute of Health Education*, 23 (1): 16–21.

Tones, K. (1990) 'Why theorise? Ideology in health education.' *Health Education Journal*, 49 (1): 2–6.

Tones, K. (1993) 'The theory of health promotion: implications for nursing', in Wilson-Barnett, J. and Macleod Clark, J. (eds) *Research in Health Promotion and Nursing*, Basingstoke: Macmillan.

Tones, K. (1997) 'Health education, behaviour change and the public health', in Detels, R., Holland, W.W., McEwen, J. and Omenn, G.S. (eds) *Oxford Textbook of Public Health* (3rd edn), Oxford: Oxford University Press.

Tones, K. (2000) 'Evaluating health promotion: a tale of three errors.' *Patient Education and Counselling*, 39: 227–36.

Tones, K. (2001) Health promotion: the empowerment imperative', in Scriven, A. and Orme, J. (eds) *Health Promotion: professional perspectives*, Basingstoke: Palgrave.

Tones, K. and Green, J. (2004) *Health Promotion: planning and strategies*, London: Sage.

Tones, K. and Tilford, S. (1994) *Health Education: effectiveness, efficiency and equity* (2nd edn), London: Chapman & Hall.

Tones, K. and Tilford, S. (2001) *Health Promotion: effectiveness, efficiency and equity* (3rd edn), London: Nelson Thornes.

Tones, K., Tilford, S. and Robinson, Y. (1990) *Health Education: effectiveness and efficiency*, London: Chapman & Hall.

Totten, C. (1992) (ed.) *Developing Quality in Health Education and Health Promotion: a manual for all those involved in the delivery of a quality service*, The Society of Health Education and Health Promotion Specialists.

Townsend, P., Davidson, N. and Whitehead, M. (1988) *Inequalities in Health: the Black Report and the health divide*, London: Pelican.

Townsend, P., Davidson, N. and Whitehead, M. (1992) *Inequalities in Health: the Black Report and the health divide*, London: Penguin.

Tuckett, D. (1979) 'Choices for health education: a sociological view', in Sutherland, I. (ed.) *Health Education: perspectives and choices*, London: George Allen & Unwin.

Turner, B.S. (1987) *Medical Power and Social Knowledge*, London: Sage.

Turner, J.M. (1987) 'Analytical theorizing', in Giddens, A. and Turner, J. (eds) *Social Theory Today*, Cambridge: Polity Press.

Twelker, P.A. (2003) 'The critical incident technique: a manual for its planning and implementation.' www.tiu.edu/psychology/Twelker/critical_incident_technique.htm (accessed 17 November 2006).

Twinn, S.F. and Lee, D.T.F. (1997) 'The practice of health education in acute care settings in Hong Kong: an exploratory study of the contribution of registered nurses.' *Journal of Advanced Nursing*, 25: 178–85.

UKCC (1986) *Project 2000: a new preparation for practice*, London: UKCC.

Ulfvarson, J., Bardage, C., Wredling, A-MR., Von Bahr, C. and Aami, J. (2007) 'Adherence to drug treatment in association with how the patient perceives care and information on drugs.' *Journal of Clinical Nursing*, 16: 141–8.

US Department of Health and Human Services (2000) *Healthy People 2010: understanding and improving health*. Rockville, IN: US Department of Health and Human Services.

Vermeire, E., Hearnshaw, H., Van Royen, J. and Denekens, J. (2001) 'Patient adherence to treatment: three decades of research. A comprehensive review.' *Journal of Clinical Pharmacy and Therapeutics*, 26: 331–42.

Visintainer, M.A. (1986) 'The nature of knowledge and theory in nursing.' *IMAGE: Journal of Nursing Scholarship*, 18 (2): 32–8.

Vuori, H. (1980) 'The medical model and the objectives of health education.' *International Journal of Health Education*, xxiii: 12–19.

Walker, L.O. (1971) 'Toward a clearer understanding of the concept of nursing theory.' *Nursing Research*, 20 (5): 428–35.

Walker, L.O. and Avant, K.C. (2005) *Strategies for Theory Construction in Nursing* (4th edn), Upper Saddle River, NJ: Pearson Prentice Hall.

Wallerstein, N. and Bernstein, E. (1998) 'Empowerment education: Freire's ideas adapted to health education.' *Health Education Quarterly*, 15 (4): 379–94.

Ward, M. (1997) 'Student nurses' perceptions of health promotion: a study.' *Nursing Standard*, 11 (24): 34–40.

Watkins, S. and Wilson, E. (1997) 'Establishing a public health nursing project.' *Nursing Standard*, 11 (36): 44–48.

Weber, M. (1971) 'The ideal type', in Thompson, K. and Tunstall, J. (eds) *Sociological perspectives*, Harmondsworth: Penguin.

Webster, G. (1989) 'Community development and health promotion: links between theory and practice.' A paper for the Public Health Alliance Symposium on 'Health For Who?' presented 15 December 1989 in London.

West, R. (2005) 'Time for a change: putting the transtheoretical (stages of change) model to rest.' *Addiction*, 100: 1036–9.

Whitehead, D. (1999a) 'The nature of health promotion in acute and community settings.' *British Journal of Nursing*, 8 (7): 463–7.

Whitehead, D. (1999b) 'The application of health promotion practice within the orthopaedic setting.' *Journal of Orthopaedic Nursing*, 3: 101–7.

Whitehead, D. (2000) 'Using mass media within health-promoting practice: a nursing perspective.' *Journal of Advanced Nursing*, 32 (4): 807–16.

Whitehead, D. (2001a) 'A stage planning programme model for health education/ health promotion practice.' *Journal of Advanced Nursing*, 36 (2): 311–20.

Whitehead, D. (2001b) 'A social cognitive model for health education/health promotion practice.' *Journal of Advanced Nursing*, 36 (3): 417–25.

Whitehead, D. (2001c) 'Health education, behavioural change and social psychology: nursing's contribution to health promotion.' *Journal of Advanced Nursing*, 34 (6): 822–32.

Whitehead, D. (2003) 'Evaluating health promotion: a model for nursing practice.' *Journal of Advanced Nursing*, 41 (5): 490–8.

Whitehead, D. (2004a) 'Health promotion and health education: advancing the concepts.' *Journal of Advanced Nursing*, 47 (3): 311–20.

Whitehead, D. (2004b) 'The European Health Promoting Hospitals (HPH) project: How far on?' *Health Promotion International*, 19 (2): 259–67.

Whitehead, D. (2005c) 'In pursuit of pleasure: health education as a means of facilitating the "health journey" of young people.' *Health Education*, 105 (3): 213–27.

Whitehead, D. (2005d) 'Health Promoting Hospitals: the role and function of nursing.' *Journal of Clinical Nursing*, 14: 20–7.

Whitehead, D. (2005a) 'The culture, context and progress of health promotion in nursing', in Scriven, A. (ed.) *Health promoting practice: the contribution of nurses and allied health professionals*. Basingstoke: Palgrave Macmillan.

Whitehead, D. (2005b) 'Letter to the editor.' *Research in nursing and health*, 28: 357–9.

Whitehead, D. (2006) 'Commentary on Irvine, F. (2005) Exploring district nursing competencies in health promotion: the use of the Delphi technique.' *Journal of Clinical Nursing*, 14: 965–75; *Journal of Clinical Nursing*, 15: 649–56.

Whitehead. D. (2007a) 'Reviewing health promotion in nursing education.' *Journal of Advanced Nursing*, 47 (3): 311–20.

Whitehead, D. (2007b) 'Health promotion and health education practice: nurses' perceptions.' *Journal of Advanced Nursing*, 61 (2): 181–7.

Whitehead, D. and Russell, G. (2004) 'How effective are health education programmes – resistance, reactance, rationality and risk? Recommendations for effective practice.' *International Journal of Nursing Studies*, 41: 163–72.

Whitehead, D., Keast, J., Montgomery, V. and Hayman, S. (2004) 'A preventive health education programme for osteoporosis.' *Journal of Advanced Nursing*, 47 (1): 15–24.

Whitehead, M. and Tones, K. (1991) *Avoiding the Pitfalls*, London: HEA.

Whitelaw, S., Baxendale, A., Bryce, C., Machardy, L., Young, I. and Witney, E. (2001) '"Settings" based health promotion: a review.' *Health Promotion International*, 16 (4): 339–53.

Whiting, L.S. (2001) 'Health promotion: the views of children's nurses.' *Paediatric Nursing*, 13 (3): 27–31.

Whittington, C. and Holland, R. (1985) 'A framework for theory in social work.' *Issues in Social Work Education*, 5 (1): 25–49.

WHO (1954) 'Expert committee on health education of the public.' First Report, WHO Technical Report Series, No. 89, Copenhagen: WHO.

WHO (1969) 'Planning and evaluation of health education services.' WHO Technical Report Series, No. 409, Copenhagen: WHO.

WHO (1978) *Declaration of Alma-Ata*. www.who.int/hpr/archive/docs/almaata.html.

WHO (1983) 'New approaches to health education in primary care.' Report of a WHO Expert Committee. WHO Technical Report Series, No. 690, Copenhagen: WHO.

WHO (1984) 'Health promotion: a WHO discussion document on the concept and principles.' Copenhagen: WHO, 9–13 July.

WHO (1985) 'Targets for health for all. Targets in support of the European regional strategy for health for all.' Copenhagen: World Health Organization Regional Office for Europe.

WHO (1986) *Ottawa Charter for Health Promotion*. www.who.int/hpr/archive/docs/ottawa.html (accessed 14 November 2007).

WHO (1991a) *The Budapest Declaration on Health Promoting Hospitals*. Budapest, 31 May–1 June.

WHO (1991b) 'Meeting global health challenges: a position paper on health education.' XIV World Conference on Health Education, Helsinki, Finland, 16–21 June.

WHO (1991c) 'Health for all targets: the health policy for Europe.' European Health for All Series, No. 4. Copenhagen: World Health Organization Regional Office for Europe.

WHO (1993) 'Health for all targets: the health policy for Europe.' European Health for All Series, No. 4, Copenhagen: WHO Regional Office for Europe.

WHO (1997a) 'Jakarta Declaration on leading health promotion into the 21st century.' The Fourth International Conference on Health Promotion: New Players for a New Era – Leading Health Promotion into the 21st Century; meeting in Jakarta, 21–25 July.

WHO (1997b) 'Health promoting hospitals: working for health, the Vienna recommendations.' Third workshop of National/Regional Health Promoting Hospitals Network Coordinators, Vienna, 16 April 1997, the Hospital Unit, WHO Regional Office for Europe.

WHO (1998a) *Health Promotion Glossary*, Geneva: World Health Organization.

WHO (1998b) *Health Promotion Evaluation: recommendations to policymakers*.

WHO (2000) *Munich Declaration: nurses and midwives: a force for health, 2000*. www.who.int/AboutWHO/Policy/20010828_4 (accessed 24 September 2007).

Wilkinson, G. and Miers, M. (1999) *Power and Nursing Practice*, Basingstoke: Macmillan.

Williams, T. (2002) 'Patient empowerment and ethical decision-making: the patient/partner and the right to act.' *Dimensions of Critical Care Nursing*, 21 (3): 100–4.

Wilson, G. (1999/2000) 'Patients know best.' *Nursing Management*, 6 (8): 18–19.

Wilson-Barnett, J. and Latter, S. (1993) 'Factors influencing nurses' health education and health promotion practice in acute ward areas', in Wilson-Barnett, J. and Macleod Clark, J. (eds) *Research in Health Promotion and Nursing*, Basingstoke: Macmillan: 61–71.

Winett, R.A. (1995) 'A framework for health promotion and disease prevention programs.' *American Psychologist*, 50 (5): 341–50.

Woolsey, L.K. (1986) 'The critical incident technique: an innovative qualitative method of research.' *Canadian Journal of Counselling*, 20 (4): 242–54.

Wright, J., Franks, A., Ayres, P., Jones, K., Roberts, T. and Whitty, P. (2002) 'Public health in hospitals: the missing link in health promotion.' *Journal of Public Health Medicine*, 24 (3): 152–5.

Wu, Tsu-Yin and Pender, N. (2005) 'A panel study of physical activity in Taiwanese youth. Testing the revised health promotion model.' *Family Community Health*, 28 (2): 113–24.

Zerwkh, J.V. (1992) 'The practice of empowerment of coercion by expert public health nurses.' *Image: Journal of Nursing Scholarship*, 24 (2): 101–5.

Zola, I. (1972) 'Medicine as an institution of social control.' *Sociological Review*, 20: 487–504.

INDEX

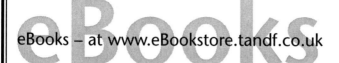